*A User's Guide to
Community Entry for the
Severely Handicapped*

SUNY Series in Special Education
David A. Sabatino, Editor

A User's Guide to Community Entry for the Severely Handicapped

ERNEST PANCSOFAR
ROBERT BLACKWELL

State University of New York Press

Published by
State University of New York Press, Albany
© 1986 State University of New York

For information, address State University of New York
Press, State University Plaza, Albany, N.Y., 12246

Library of Congress Cataloging in Publication Data

Panscofar, Ernest
    A user's guide to community entry for the severely
handicapped.
(SUNY series in special education)
Bibliography: p.
Includes index.
1. Handicapped—Housing—United States. 2. Group
homes for the handicapped—United States. 3. Halfway
houses—United States. I. Blackwell, Robert.
II. Title. III. Series.
HV156.2U5P36 1985   362.4′0485′0973   84-
HV156.2U5P36 1985   362.4′0485′0973   84-24139
ISBN 0-88706-034-X
ISBN 0-88706-035-8 (pbk.)

10 9 8 7 6 5 4 2 1 1

To

The late Mrs. Pearl Granger who dedicated most of her life to providing residential homes for exceptional individuals.

and

The residents of the John Collier House in Eugene, Oregon, for the experiences they provided.

Contents

Preface

A DECADE AGO there would not have been interest, and
therefore little reason, to prepare a guide directed at entering
individuals with severe handicaps into independent living. In the
previous decade, following the advent of the Pennsylvania Decision
(1971), the rights of all mentally retarded persons as citizens were
finally questioned. The response was an increased intensity in
awareness, first for a few select parents and professionals, growing
till now many have had some direct experience in the process of
preparing individuals with handicaps for competitive employment
and independent living, to the degree which they can profit.

State schools and hospitals across this land have changed
dramatically in the past five years. These institutions oddly enough,
were begun under the influence of European nurturists in the late
18th century to provide a cure for mental retardation. When that cure
was not realized, hope deminished and by the beginning of the 20th
century, institutions for the mentally retarded were no longer aimed
at normalization or redirected human development, but at becoming
warehouses of humanity. Indeed, mounds, if not mountains of
relatively undifferentiated subnormal individuals by definition,
became scrap heaps, without hope or any thought of a long range goal
that would remove them from within their institutional walls. Many
came there as infants, and left there on the way to interment. If they
were very well behaved, and learned quickly, relatively speaking, they
raked leaves, swept floors, and did other meaningless activities.

Breakthroughs in other countries, Sweden's communal hostels, the Russian denial of genetic mental retardation, and observations in this country in some of the better administered jobs and life oriented programs brought an awareness that more could be done.

With the work of the Pennsylvania Association for Retarded Citizens, the Parsons (Kansas) Groups, the Group at the Columbia State School and Hospital, the Kennedy Centers, Wisconsin Central Colony, and a number of dedicated professional forerunners (Baumeister, Blatt, Warren, Brown, and many many others), the educable or mild groups of mentally retarded disappeared from the state schools entirely. The moderate group filled into the education classes they left, and the severe and profoundly mentally retarded were literally lifted from rubber lined mattresses and from rocking chairs on sun porches and given the right to learn to do for themselves. Today, vocational related behaviors and the range of skills needed to approximate independent living are being taught in a systematic manner.

To the audience of parents, paraprofessionals, community or institutional volunteers, professionals from a wide range of disciplines interested in planning community entry and independent living skills, Pancsofar and Blackwell have constituted an easily read, step-by-step approach, with few assumptions. To the administrator considering some type of community living, to their boards, this book is most aptly suited. It approaches the topic of alternative living as a plan, a road map, a user's guide, with procedural steps, and concepts for the decision maker.

Chapter One begins with no elaborate warm up as it probes the reader's level of awareness and commitment. It is obvious that these authors understand the necessity of commitment. They bring the reader the concepts of normalization, criteria of ultimate functioning, the competence-deviance hypothesis, least restrictive environment, dignity of risk, and ecological orientation. The next two chapters examine housing and community living options. The next chapter looks at financial concerns. Chaper 5 looks at the transition in moving residents. Chapter 6 examines the necessity and development of voluntary community resources. Chapter 7 provides a range of instructional strategies for staff members within residential settings. Chapters 8, 9, and 10 delineate several parameters within the life functioning areas of domestic living, leisure pursuits, and general community functioning. Finally, Chapter 11 concludes with a discussion of the authors' list of characteristics that differentiates model training efforts within residential settings.

Who should read this user's guide? Anyone interested in programming, planning for, and investing in residential and community living for persons with severe handicaps. Why? Because under one cover, the authors have raised and answered, with specific step-by-step precision, the predominate questions for the successful entry of these individuals into residential options which require a growing approximation toward total independence.

David A. Sabatino
Menomonie, Wisconsin

Introduction

T HE INTENT of this text is to provide guidelines for developing comprehensive residential options for individuals who are severely handicapped. Persons with severe handicaps are characterized by physical or mental impairments or conditions that place them at a disadvantage in a major life activity such as ambulation, communication, self-care, socialization, vocational training, employment, transportation, adapting to housing, etc.. Severe handicaps are those physical or mental impairment or condition that are static, of long duration, or slowly progressive (Office of Information and Resources of the Handicapped of the Department of Education).

Residential planning board members need to develop systematic strategies for insuring that all members of the community, regardless of the severity of the handicapping condition, be allowed to live in a setting as homelike as possible. By following the guidelines that are outlined in subsequent chapters, direct care staff members and administrative personnel will find useful recommendations for achieving the goal of residential placement in the least restrictive environment for residents with severely handicapping conditions. Adherence to these recommendations requires a commitment by residential personnel to acknowledge the rights of all citizens to live in their home community. Along with this commitment is an obligation to develop residential alternatives that match the unique characteristics of individuals with severe handicaps to home environments that foster as great a degree of independence as possible.

Chapter 1

Philosophic Orientation

T HIS TEXT BEGINS with a discussion of the motivational
influences that are found in well-organized, resident-oriented
agencies that provide a full range of home-living experiences. Each
agency possesses a character or set of values that are perceived by
public and professional persons alike. The development and
operation of a set of values or philosophic orientation is a necessary
first step in providing the framework for a quality existence for
individuals with severe handicaps.

A philosophy of operation is a set of *guiding principles* that forms the
underlying reasons why we function as we do with individuals with
severely handicapping conditions. Even beyond our work in this
human service area "a central guiding principle is needed in all human
activities." (Dubos, 1981, p 202) Schumacher (1973) emphasizes this
orientation:

> All subjects, no matter how specialized, are connected with a centre;
> they are like rays emanating from the sun. The centre is constituted by
> our most basic convictions, by those ideas which really have the power to
> move us. (p. 94)

In relation to community planning of residential options for
persons with severe handicaps, what are these rays made of? The
following philosophic orientations will be highlighted in this opening
chapter as representing the current guiding principles in residential
planning for persons with severe handicaps.

- Normalization

- Criterion of Ultimate Functioning
- Competence-Deviance Hypothesis
- Least Restrictive Environment
- Dignity of Risk
- Ecological Orientation

Figure 1 contains an illustration of how Schumacher (1973) might have envisioned the previously enumerated philosophic orientations as they emanate from a core area of each person's inner convictions.

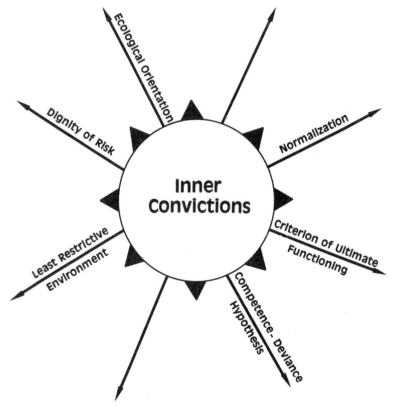

At the core of our imaginary sun are our personal beliefs, convictions, commitments and priorities, that alter the operation of surrounding rays of light. We must begin with our own personal changes, convictions, and goals before we attempt to guide other people's lives; especially the lives of residents who are severely handicapped. For change to occur we must begin with ourselves (Blatt, 1981; Buscaglia, 1982). "Before I ask the world to change, I must change. I am the beginning step." (Blatt, 1981, p. 12)

One man, greatly respected by Burton Blatt, was Dick Hungerford who wrote a beautiful essay commemorating the first meeting of
the then National Association for Retarded Children (circa. 1950).
The following is a quote from this presentation:

> My office window looks out on a near-tenement street. In the main
> there are curtains awry at the windows; there are rusted fire escapes
> with half-filled milk bottles precariously perched on them. The pavement
> is littered with papers, listlessly moving in the March dusk. And at the
> end of the street there is Bellevue, a city hospital. In general it is not
> pleasant.
> Two apartments, however, are different. The same kind of fire
> escape breaks the view; the same dirty pavement is beneath. But in these
> apartments the windows are clean, the curtains are starched and white,
> the Venetian blinds are evenly drawn. And a light has been lit. They have
> met a common problem and found dignity.
> So I think it must be with each one of us. This is our street. We can
> be ruined by it, or we can bring meaning to it and to ourselves.
> And perhaps that is the sameness for which our hearts long. All
> streets have grayness, at one end of every street there is a Bellevue. All
> problems are difficult, it is always hard to work in the half-light, the
> partially understood, which encompasses so much of living. We cannot
> run away from life. We cannot pick up all the empty milk bottles or
> isolate all the derelicts. We must not judge harshly Man-or God. We
> must be kindly. We must work with everything that we have for the
> betterment of the street where we are placed. And we must keep
> our windows clean and turn on the lights against the common twilight.
> (Hungerford, 1950, p. 418)

The main question becomes: How do I become the best person
that I am capable of becoming in order to affect more positively the
lives of people I come in contact with?

Three suggestions are provided to begin the process of solidifying
our inner convictions.

First, we must acknowledge that what each of us perceive in the
world around us are approximations of what is really there. We all
possess uniquely different sensory perceptors and process information at different speeds and with different background references to
evaluate this input. Therefore, no one can claim to have all the
answers on any given topic. Michel (1981) relates that "For every
expert, there's an equal and opposite expert." We need to begin
thinking less in dichotomies (either-or) and more in combinations of
relationships that are possible when evaluating a particular problem.
Thus, the first proposition is to consent that none of us know the
truth, but we may be able to lay claims on approximations of the Truth
as we perceive it to be.

Secondly, each of us needs to keep a personal journal. Included in a journal are thoughts about various events you've experienced during the day, observations, uncollected thoughts, excerpts from books that have had a positive impact, creative manipulations of ideas, setting goals and priorities (of both short and long duration). In essence, it's a written communication to oneself expressing thoughts that ordinarily would not resurface without confronting them again days, weeks, or years later in a journal. A journal should be a chronology of growth toward resolving issues of both philosophic and pragmatic origin.

Third, we must actively participate in discussions of ethical dimensions. Sample topic areas might include:

• What is the role of a profoundly mentally retarded member of society?
• What happen after we die? (You may not be right, but this perception provides a catalyst for existing choices.)
• How do you feel toward parents of severely handicapped students?
• What are your feelings on terminating a pregnancy when it's known that the unborn child will have Down's Syndrome?
• Why do bad things happen to good people?

These are just a few topics that should be discussed in college courses and residential in-services that are preparing persons to work with individuals with severe handicaps.

A detailed explanation now follows addressing the prevailing philosophic principles that appear to be at the forefront of the residential movement for the severely handicapped. The day-to-day operation of these guiding principles will be affected by each individual's personal beliefs and inner convictions.

Normalization

Wolfensberger (1972) is the author who is given credit for expanding the principle of normalization from previously enunciated definitions by Bank-Mikkelsen and Nirje from the Scandanavian countries. Recently, Wolfensberger (1980) offered the following revision:

> The use of means which are culturally normative to offer a person life conditions at least as good as the average citizen's and to as much as possible enhance or support personal behaviors, appearances, status, and reputation to the greatest degree possible at any given time for

each individual according to his or her development needs.

Nirjie (1977) very beautifully incorporates eight basic tenets of normalization into the following poem:

Normalization means... a normal rhythm of the day.
You get out of bed in the morning, even if you are profoundly retarded and physically handicapped;
you get dressed,
and leave the house for school or work, you don't stay home;
in the morning you anticipate events,
in the morning you think back on what you have accomplished;
the day is not a monotonous 24 hours with every minute endless.
You eat at normal times of the day and in a normal fashion;
not just with a spoon, unless you are an infant;
not in bed, but at a table;
not early in the afternoon for the convenience of the staff.

Normalization means ... a normal rhythm of the week.
You live in one place,
go to work in another,
and participate in leisure activities in yet another.
You anticipate leisure activities on weekends,
and look forward to getting back to school or work on Monday.

Normalization...a normal rhythm of the year.
A vacation to break the routineness of the year.
Seasonal changes bring with them a variety of types of food, work, cultural events, sports, leisure activities.
Just think...we thrive on these seasonal changes.

Normalization means...normal developmental experiences of the life cycle.
In childhood, children, but not adults, go to summer camps.
In adolescence, one is interested in grooming, hair styles, music, boyfriends, and girlfriends.
In adulthood, life is filled with work and responsibilities.
In old age, one has memories to look back on, and can enjoy the wisdom of experience.

Normalization means...having a range of choices, wishes, and desires respected and considered.
Adults have the freedom to decide
where they would like to live,
what kind of job they would like to have, and can best perform.
Whether they would prefer to go bowling with a group, instead of staying home to watch television.

Normalization means...living in a world made of two sexes.
Children and adults both develop relationships with members of the

opposite sex.
Teenagers become interested in having boyfriends and girlfriends.
And adults may fall in love, and decide to marry.

Normalization means...the right to normal economic standards.
All of us have basic financial privileges and responsibilities.
are able to take advantage of compensatory economic security means,
    such as child allowances, old age pensions, and minimum wage
    regulation.
We should have money to decide how to spend; on personal luxuries or
    necessities.

Normalization means...living in normal housing in a normal neigh-
    borhood.
Not in a large facility with 20, 50, or 100 other people because you are
    retarded.
And not isolated from the rest of the community.
Normal locations and normal size homes will give residents better
    opportunities for successful integration within their communities.

Additionally, included in the *Way to Go* publication is a list of eight
"clangers" associated with normalization. A "clanger" is an internal
bell that should signal to us that an observed situation is counter to
the principle of normalization.

Clangers

1. Does what we see seem to fit the circumstances?
2. Is what we see appropriate for us? For our children?
3. Would something we see make us feel strange or out of place
   if it were happening to us?
4. What image is probably conveyed to others by what we see?
5. Does what we see give evidence of growth, warmth, and
   caring?
6. Would we like to live there, work there, play there?
7. Could we improve what we see?
8. Can we think of a better way to do it? (Cooney, 1978).

In summary, normalization is a modus operandi, the backbone of
our relationship with individuals with severely handicapping
conditions. It is an often abused term when merely renaming cottages
and rearranging furniture is the extent of an adherence to a
normalization philosophy (McCord, 1982). Normalization can be a
powerful defense toward developing more acceptable and enlightened
interactions with "different functioning" individuals.

Criterion of Ultimate Functioning

The criterion of ultimate functioning was a phrase coined by Brown, Nietupski, and Hamre-Nietupski (1976) and "...refers to the ever changing expanding localized, and personalized cluster of factors that each person must possess in order to function as productively and independently as possible in socially, vocationally, and domestically integrated community environments." (p. 11)

Eight questions emerge from the above statement relating to the choice of activities for severely handicapped residents.

The Value of Certain Instructional Practices

1. Why should we engage in this activity?
2. Is this activity necessary to prepare residents to ultimately function in complex heterogeneous community settings?
3. Could residents function as adults if they did not acquire the skill?
4. Is there a different activity that will allow residents to approximate realization of the criterion of ultimate functioning more quickly and more efficiently?
5. Will this activity impede, restrict or reduce the probability that residents will ultimately function in community settings?
6. Are the skills, materials, tasks, and criteria of concern similar to those encountered in adult life?

Competence-Deviance Hypothesis

Gold (1980) proposes that the more competence an individual has, the more deviance will be tolerated in him/her by others. He describes deviance as those aspects of an individual which cause negative attention. He describes competence as those attributes and skills which not everyone has, and which are appreciated and needed by someone else.

We all have some unique, deviant behavior but we can readily distinguish private from public environments. Some of our behaviors would cause negative attention if observed outside the confines of our home, i.e., eating habits, behavior while viewing a sports event or singing loudly in the shower are but a few examples.

Let's take a look at potential deviant behavior and how it can be acceptable in one situation and unacceptable under a different set of circumstances. Marc Gold was a human being who was eminently respected in and out of the field of Special Education because of his immense contributions to his discipline. Marc Gold also wore his hair in a pony tail and had a very pronounced moustache. If Dr. Gold had decided to make a midlife career change and seek a job as a salesperson for Xerox or IBM, these same physical attributes would not be tolerated. In other words, his competence would not be of such a magnitude that his deviant (negative attention) behavior would be tolerated.

Another example of dubious deviance is chewing tobacco and spitting. To many people, this is obnoxious behavior but when the manager of a recent world series baseball team is seen on national television exhibiting this deviant behavior, it is easily tolerated. His competent behavior far overshadowed behavior which did cause negative attention from some baseball fans...but it was tolerated!

How do the above two examples relate to residents who are severely handicapped? These residents display many behaviors which are apt to evoke negative reactions from people, i.e., drooling, incontinence, lack of mobility, hand flapping, etc. Our task as trainers is not to rid each resident of all deviant behavior (that would be impossible!), but to enable that individual to possess competent behavior so that the remaining deviant behavior will be more tolerated by others. Examples of competence can range from learning how to be an excellent swimmer or being able to assemble a complex circuitry board to the ability to be pleasant when someone is talking to you (this behavior is surely valued and appreciated and certainly something not everyone has).

Least Restrictive Environment

The derivation of the concept of the least restrictive alternative will be discussed as it relates to residential placement for persons with severe handicaps. In the area of mental health, the first legal opinion addressing this concept occurred in 1966 in the *Lake v. Cameron* court of appeals decision. Mrs. Cameron had been committed to a mental hospital because of a history of wandering away from her home. In the opinion of the court, less restrictive means could have been employed by the state without resorting to commitment. Examples of less restrictive alternatives mentioned in this opinion included the use of an indentification card, public health nursing care, and foster care (Mickenberg, 1980). Six years later, Judge Johnson, in *Wyatt v. Stickney,* defined the least restrictive alternative as including the movement of residents from: (a) more to less structured living, (b) larger to smaller facilities, (c) larger to smaller living units, (d) group to individual residence, (e) segregated from the community to integrated into community living, and (f) dependent to independent living.

The previous two court decisions, in conjunction with several similar opinions throughout the country, paved the way for Section 504 of P.L. 93-112. Often cited as a mandate for the right of all persons with handicaps to live in the least restrictive environment, Section 504 states that:

> No otherwise qualified handicapped individual in the United States shall, solely by reason of his handicap, be excluded from participation, be denied the benefits of, or be subjected to discrimination under any program or activity, receiving federal financial assistance.

Laski (1980) concludes that as a result of the language of Section 504, the committee proceedings concerning the law, the history of related enactments, its administrative construction, and several judicial opinions that Section 504: (a) required that the segregation of disabled people be ended, (b) prohibited unnecessary separate services and required that services be provided in the most integrated settings, (c) required that disabled people be admitted equally to all services and to the equal benefit of all services, and (d) required that disabled people be provided services equally effective as those provided to the general population.

An additional statement concerning the least restrictive alternative can be found in the Developmentally Disabled Assistance and Bill of Rights Act of 1975. In part, this law "...provides that persons with developmental disabilities have a right to appropriate treatment, services, and habilitation for such disabilities...(services) should be designed to maximize the developmental potential of the person and should be provided in the setting that is least restrictive of the person's personal liberty."

The previous statements from court opinions and federal laws do not contain adequate descriptions for defining the parameters of the concept of a least restrictive alternative. Many members of human service planning agencies interpret the least restrictive alternative as options available, possible, and/or economically feasible. For example, if options that are available within a community are only considered, the range would be extremely limited for communities with few resources. A small town of 12,000 may presently not have a group home and, therefore, suggest placement in a regional residential center as an available option for a severely handicapped person. However, if that same town had a planning agency whose members chose to interpret the concept as the least restrictive alternative possible, they would encourage the development of residential options within the community that would provide a living environment for all handicapped residents based on their current functioning level. There are also planning agencies whose members will weigh the pros and cons of residential placement by using a financial yard stick for determining the least restrictive alternative. Often these agency members are swayed by cost-benefit information that is not derived from a common denominator and thus provides an inaccurate comparison.

Dignity of Risk

Perske (1972) expressed the essence of a dignity of risk orientation in his article in *Mental Retardation:*

> You are a human being and so you have the right to live as other humans live, even to the point where we will not take all dangers of human life from you.
> [There is a] human dignity in risk and there can be a dehumanizing indignity in safety.

In his definition of a dignity of risk, Perske is not advocating a reckless abandon approach in our interactions with persons who have severe handicaps. Instead, he is recommending that we challenge these residents and give them skills to become adaptable and autonomous when they enter adult service options. Risks are a normal daily occurrence in crossing streets at busy intersections, playing on the public park's recreation equipment, learning a skilled vocational occupation, camping and outdoor leisure pursuits.

In relation to the previously enumerated activities, individuals with severe handicaps must be adequately prepared and demonstrate relevant safety behaviors. For example, if a resident does not respond to the verbal cue "stop" in a training setting, it would be foolish to immediately allow him/her to walk unassisted in a busy parking lot where a car might unexpectedly cross the student's path while the teacher is giving a cue "stop." There is a definite line that needs to be distinguished between acceptable risk and foolheartiness. Of specific concern is the student's mobility, physical stature, response to verbal safety cues, auditory and visual acuity, and tolerance level under multiple stimulus conditions.

ECOLOGICAL ORIENTATION

Russell (1976) in his book *Health Education,* strongly advocates for an ecological orientation to a decision-making process. "Relationships to understand" should replace a "problem to solve" attitude by persons responsible for decisions that affect another's present and future activities. This "relationship to understand" orientation contains four major interconnected elements: the individual, significant others, the physical environments, and culture. Pertinent information that should be included in these elements follow.

Individual
Medical Information
Psychological Reports
General likes and dislikes
Role expectations: student, worker, son/daughter, friend
Aptitudes, strengths
Primary and secondary Reinforcers

Significant Others

Primary home care giver(s)
Trainers, aides, schoolmates, therapists
Friends, peers, and siblings
Community Service Personnel

Physical Environment

School setting: classroom and grounds
Community Activity Sites
Classroom Materials
Home environment and neighborhood

Culture

Operationalized philosophic orientation of the school/community
Portrayal of handicapped persons by community news media
General attitude of nonhandicapped members toward persons
   with handicaps
Outcome of judicial and legislative decisions
Orientation of helping professionals

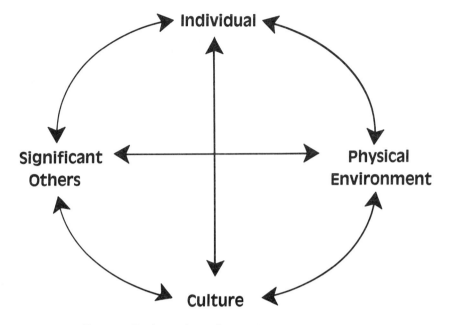

Fig. 1.2 Ecological Analysis of Decision Making

The major concept of the ecological analysis toward decision making is the impact that a change in one element has on the entire system of elements. Every element is intrinsically related to all the others. To operationalize this orientation, we would suggest that each resident have an outline of the ecological model at the front of his/her Individualized Habilitation Plan (IHP) folder. Within each model, all the pertinent information would be listed beneath each element and updated as changes occur in each element. The decision-making process must be concerned with the overall change that can be anticipated when altering one of the element's components. For example, the decision of when to initiate a toileting program for a resident cannot be made in isolation. Knowledge of the support in the home environment and of the specific individuals who can be targeted to implement the regimen must exist. More specifically, it is highly recommended that detailed inventories of skills be recorded in physical environments frequented by the resident's peers. The trainer can then assess the resident on his/her ability to independently perform as many of these skills as possible and target areas for individualized goals and objectives.

In summary, consider the effects a decision to implement a

program will have on each of the elements within the ecological model. Residential trainers must be proactive and not reactive to crises that often occur through lack of careful planning and foresight.

SUMMARY

Included in the previous sections were six guiding principles or philosophy statements with some explanatory information for each principle. How a group of community service providers operationalize these principles can be diverse. For example, two operation statements originate from The Association for Persons with Severe Handicaps (TASH—formerly, The Association for the Severely Handicapped) and the Center for Human Policy at Syracuse University.

The TASH Board of Directors passed the following resolution at its 1980 national conference:

> To realize the goals and objectives of The Association for the Severely Handicapped, the following resolution is adopted: In order to develop, learn, grow and live as fully as possible, persons with handicapping conditions require access to services which allow for longitudinal, comprehensive, systematic and chronological age appropriate interactions with persons without identified handicaps. Such interactions must occur in domestic living, educational, vocational and recreational/leisure environments. Specifically, handicapped individuals should: 1) participate in family-like and/or normalized community-based domestic living environments; 2) receive educational services in chronological age appropriate regular educational environments; 3) receive training in and access to a wide variety of vocational environments and opportunities, regardless of functioning level; and 4) participate in a wide range of normalized recreational/leisure environments and activities that involve persons without identified handicaps. The Association for the Severely Handicapped believes that the above conditions must be met in order to provide quality service and that these conditions can only be met by community-based services. Therefore, The Association for the Severely Handicapped resolves that it will work toward the rapid termination of living environments and educational/vocational/recreational services that segregate, regiment and isolate persons from the individualized attention and sustained normalized community interactions necessary for maximal growth, development and the enjoyment of life.

Similarly, Bogdan (1979) issued the following statement in a widely disseminated manuscript:

In the domain of Human Rights:

All people have fundamental moral and constitutional rights. These rights must not be abrogated merely because a person has a mental or physical disability.
Among these fundamental rights is the right to community living.

In the domain of Educational Programming and Human Service:

All people, as human beings are inherently valuable.
All people can grow and develop.
All people are entitled to conditions which foster their development.
Such conditions are optimally provided in community settings.

Therefore:

In fulfillment of fundamental human rights and
In securing optimum developmental opportunities,
all people, regardless of the severity of their disabilities, are entitled to community living.

There are many approaches available for changing the life options of severely handicapped individuals. An organization may not feel that the strongly worded statements from TASH or Bogdan (1979) best personify the intent of its charter and may present their own statement of operation. An organization functions at a higher level of efficiency when its members know the underlying philosophic principles for its day-to-day actions. Six guiding principles have been detailed in this chapter. Without a personal commitment that is based on one or more of these principles, the following chapters will not assist individuals to facilitate the entry of persons with severe handicaps into the community.

Chapter 2

Range of Residential Options

THE PURPOSE of this chapter is to describe a range of possible living environments for persons with severely handicapping conditions. Additionally, a brief look at the present controversy on the means of enabling residents to live in the least restrictive environment possible will be explored.

Community Living Alternatives

The following list contains a variety of living arrangements with their respective brief definitions. The list is not to be evaluated as an attempt to place options in a least to most restricted nature or most preferred to least preferred. This decision must be made after evaluating the unique circumstances of each resident.

1. **Independent Living:** A site where an individual lives with a roommate, a spouse, or alone; usually an apartment or duplex, but occasionally a house.
   Single-Family Homes: A free standing single-family home in an average residential neighborhood. (4)
   Shared Homes: Two or more handicapped persons may prefer to share a single-family home and the cost of needed modification—often the sharing is between handicapped and congenial, able-bodied persons (4)

Individual or Shared Apartments: In large or small buildings, apartments occupied by a single handicapped person, or shared by two or more, have been used successfully with or without services, depending on need. (4)

Groups of Individual Apartments: Groups of apartments—on one floor or scattered throughout the building or scattered among several buildings in an apartment complex. (4)

Dwellings in New Apartment Buildings: Some percentage of the living units in a large public or private apartment building can be designed for the handicapped. (4)

Elderly Housing Projects: Projects for the elderly that are designed with special facilities may have a percentage of the units set aside for the handicapped, with provision of the additional services needed. (4)

Congregate Housing: A residential environment—assisted independent living—that incorporates shelter and services for the functionally impaired and/or marginally socially adjusted elderly or handicapped persons, enabling them to maintain or return to a semi-independent lifestyle and avoid institutionalization. (4)

Residential Hotels: Relatively large structures that provide private rooms and baths (not apartments) are adaptable for the handicapped, with housekeeping and meal service available at commercial rates. (4)

2. **Natural or Adoptive Home:** The home of one's parents, usually natural parents. (2)

3. **Other Relative's Home:** The home of a resident's sibling, grandparent, aunt, uncle, or offspring. (2)

4. **Friend's Home:** The home of someone who has befriended the resident or the resident's family. (2)

5. **Foster Family Care:** Serving five or fewer retarded adults in a family's own home, families are not governed by board of directors, and they collect monthly payments for the care of residents. (1)

6. **Developmental Foster Home:** Similar to natural homes, foster homes, and adoptive homes, these homes should offer a living situation to a child that encourages a sense of identity and security in a homelike setting for up to three children. Placements are often made with the expressed objective that a child will remain with his developmental foster family until he/she reaches adulthood. Developmental foster home parents are trained to extend the services of the developmental center or public school program into the home environment. (3)

7. **Group Homes:** Homes that house as few as two or as many as 100 developmentally disabled children or adults. (2)

   Five or more handicapped persons of both sexes may live in a relatively large home (purchased, rented, or constructed), assisted by house managers or counselors and providing access to any other services, internal and external required. (4)

   Small Group Home: serving 10 or fewer retarded adults. (2)

   Medium Group Home: serving 11 to 20 retarded adults. (2)

   Large Group Home: serving 21 to 40 retarded adults. (2)

   Mini-institution: serving 41 to 80 retarded adults. (2)

   Mixed Group Home: serving retarded adults and former mental hospital patients and/or ex-offenders in the same residence. (2)

   Group Home for Older Adults: serving only older retarded people and often nonretarded people as well in group homes or rest homes. (2)

8. **Nursing Homes:** Include a variety of residential alternatives, all providing continuing medical care for anyone who needs it. The convalescent home and intermediate care facility are specially licensed nursing homes. Nursing homes are nearly always privately owned and are expected to make a profit for their owners. (2)

   Intermediate Care Facilities (ICF): Licensed as a nursing home, making it eligible for Federal Medicaid Support (Title XIX) of The Social Security Act and its Amendments). Two classes are distinguished according to size: 15 and under, and 16 and over. The larger homes must have a nurse (LPN) on duty at all times, whereas the smaller homes need only have one on call. (2)

   Convalescent Homes: A nursing home whose residents are expected to stay for a reasonably short period of time for rehabilitation before they return to the community. (2)

   The County Home: type of nursing home whose residents are expected to stay for a reasonably short period of time for rehabilitation before they return to the community. (2)

9. **Boarding Homes:** Homes where the resident is provided room and board for a fee, but no other services are contracted. These homes house individuals of varying abilities. They are usually not classified as group or family care homes. (2)

10. **Hostel:** Similar to residential hotel but a hostel is usually supervised and is considered transitional or temporary. (4)

11. **Sheltered Villages:** Provide a segregated, self-contained community for retarded adults and live-in staff in a cluster of buildings usually located in a rural setting. (1)

12. **Public Residential Facility** (PRF): State institutions. Until recently these were very large, typically having about 1,500 residents and occasionally having over 5,000, but today they average only about 500 residents each, and many have fewer than 50. (2)
13. **Private Residential Facility:** A variety of privately-owned and foundation-owned residential alternatives. Some of these are expensive, highly visible, multiple-treatment centers, some are largely custodial facilities, and some are communes that feature an idyllic life for handicapped and nonhandicapped co-residents. (2)
14. **Workshop-Dormitories:** Living unit and a work training program are associated administratively and sometimes physically. (1)
15. **Mental Hospital:** An institution for mentally ill individuals. (2)
16. **Prisons:** A building, usually with cells, where convicted criminals are confined or where accused persons are held while awaiting trial. (5)

> 1 = Baker, Seltzer, & Seltzer (1977)
> 2 = Heal, Novak, Sigelman, & Switzky (1980)
> 3 = Lensink (1980)
> 4 = Thompson (1977)
> 5 = Webster (1980)

A primary living environment for children and young adolescents would be to enable them to reside within the natural family (option #2). There are a multitude of personal reasons why parents choose to place a child with severe handicaps outside the home setting. Many revolve around marriage crises, sibling unrest, financial concerns, and lack of support from relatives and community helping professionals. Lensink (1980) provides the following incentives for enhancing the prospects of a family retaining a child within the home:

- trained child-care providers
- parent consultations
- training in speech, motor, and sensory development
- behavior management
- residential respite
- housekeeping assistance
- crisis medical and behavior problem assistance teams
- trained companions for handicapped teens

- advocacy and assistance with generic health, education, and rehabilitation services agencies
- family counseling
- behavior therapy and psychotherapy for nonhandicapped family members
- direct subsidization of costs of caring for a handicapped person

Parents should be contacted by area Associations for Retarded Citizens, Council for Exceptional Children, university student and professional organizations, local advocacy groups, local chapters of the Association for Persons with Severe Handicaps and other helping organizations to secure many of Lensink's (1980) recommendations.

During adolescence or as a young adult, individuals should be encouraged to explore additional living environments. This exploration need not occur on a permanent basis. For example Freagen, Wheeler, Hill, Brankin, and Costello (1982) recommend that as part of the secondary education plan for adolescents with severe handicaps, brief 2-3 day overnight stays in a group home setting would allow for instruction in real, subsequent living environments.

The choice of where an individual should reside is not a clear-cut issue. The range in quality of any of the options is extremely diverse. For example, even though placement of a child or adolescent within the home environment is of primary concern, not all parents provide a caring atmosphere and unfortunately, child abuse and neglect are not isolated occurrences. Additionally, a small group home of up to five residents may be operated in such a manner that more restrictions could occur than in other living arrangements. Perhaps the most appropriate placement option for individuals with severe handicaps lies in an ecological analysis of variables effecting each person's life. (See Chapter One for a review of the elements within this analysis.)

Two examples follow that contain a discussion of residential options and how they can be analyzed from an ecological perspective.

Evaluative Review of Sheltered Villages

A sheltered village is a rural community whose inhabitants include handicapped and nonhandicapped persons. Baker, Seltzer, and Seltzer (1977) explain that "common to all sheltered villages is the segregation of the retarded person (and often the live-in staff) from the outside community, and the implicit view that the retarded adult is better off in an environment that shelters him or her from many of the potential failures and frustrations of life in the outside community" (p 109). It is common to find a religious undertone in many sheltered villages with five of the nine surveyed by Baker, et al. (1977) being church sponsored. There were also an average of thirty-nine residents per village with a staff-to-resident ratio of 1:1.7.

Often there is controversy about adherence to the principle of normalization within sheltered villages. Some proponents of sheltered villages (particularly parents) do not feel handicapped persons need to be confronted with the crime, noise, ridicule, and other normal experiences they may contact in a community setting. Blatt (1980) relates the following anecdote about his experience within a sheltered village. One morning Blatt awoke at 5:00 a.m. and walked to the barn. At the barn he observed one resident already up and milking the cow. A second resident was holding the cow's tail. Thinking this to be a somewhat comical sight, Blatt related his observation to the director. Upon hearing Blatt's story, the director stated that the young man was performing a very useful function in the milking process by holding the tail and not allowing it to get into the milk. Blatt recalled the many times he had toured large institutions where similarly functioning persons were holding pieces of string, belts, clothes, etc. in a very nonfunctional manner. Yet in the sheltered village, a person could hold the cow's tail and provide a useful service as part of the milking process. Thus, the adherence of a sheltered village to a principle of normalization can be interpreted from several positions.

The sheltered village examined in this section is Camphill Village, Copake, New York. Camphill Village can trace its roots to Rudolph Steiner's philosophy for an equal emphasis on body, soul, and spiritual growth (anthroposophy). Modeled after Botton Village in England, Camphill Village contains a unique approach of providing residential, educational, and spiritual training for its residents (Baker, et al., 1977). At the time Baker, et al. (1977) described Camphill Village, there were 175 villagers: ninety retarded adults, forty-nine staff members, and thirty-six dependents of staff members. Staff members were unpaid workers who had either made long-term commitments to the Village or time-limited stays such as college work-study students. Residents of Camphill Village were mostly mildly retarded with approximately thirty-three percent being moderately-severely retarded. There was a strong emphasis on work and leisure activities and little effort was made to integrate villagers into a larger outside community. All work activities were assigned by the Works Group on the basis of what was needed in the Village. Leisure activities included such diverse activities as hobby groups, music, dramatic productions, folk dancing, or lectures and self-interest groups.

If an ecological analysis approach is used to determine an

A Users Guide To Community
Entry for the severely
Handicapped. (1986).
Pancsofar, Ernest. and
Blackwell, Robert.

adherence to a least restrictive alternative concept the issues of separation and protection immediately surface. The cultural element is guided by the anthroposophical works of Steiner. The key ingredients of anthroposophy are the blending of Eastern philosophical ideas with Western Christianity (Baker, et al., 1977). There is no strong emphasis toward espousing a normalization philosophy as developed by Wolfensberger (1972). Thus, the spiritual component within the cultural element of the ecological model determines the relationships of the individual, significant others, and the physical environment. If one agrees with a separate but equal philosophy, Camphill Village would rate high as a service delivery model. However, if normalization is the prevailing attitude, a sheltered village residential option would rate low on a least restrictive alternative continuum. This low rating would especially be warranted because one of the major corollaries of normalization is physical and social integration within the community.

The philosophic component aside, sheltered villages differ dramatically in training excellence. Camphill Village is an example of a well-run, integrated network of work training, leisure, and spiritual activities.

Evaluative Review of Small Group Homes

O'Connor (1976) described the average community residential facility as a large house located in the residential section of a town and within walking distance of stores and community services. Housing options of this description are generally called group homes. More specifically, Baker et al. (1977) describe six categories of group homes including: (a) small group homes — serving ten or fewer handicapped persons, (b) medium group homes — serving eleven to twenty handicapped persons, (c) large group homes — serving twenty-one to forty handicapped persons, (d) mini-institutions — serving forty-one to eighty handicapped persons, (e) mixed group homes — serving handicapped persons and former hospital patients and/or ex-offenders in the same residence, and (f) group homes for older adults — serving older handicapped persons and often nonhandicapped persons as well in group homes or rest homes.

In this section small group homes (ten or fewer) will be discussed. The purpose of a small group home is to provide persons with severe handicaps a residential environment that closely resembles a normal family unit. Group homes are often administered by public or private nonprofit associations and operated with live-in managers and/or hourly shift-staff. Live-in staff members are usually a married couple who receive room and board and a small monthly salary to provide supervision and training for the handicapped residents. Shift-staff are assigned work slots to provide supervision and training in the areas of self-help, recreation/leisure, socialization, communication, etc. The example group home delivery system detailed in this section is from Teaching Research in Monmouth, Oregon (Fredericks, Baldwin, Heyer, Romer, Romer, Gage, Vladimiroff & Johnson, 1979; Gage, Fredericks, Baldwin, Grove & Moore, 1977).

Teaching Research received a grant from the Bureau of Education for the Handicapped in 1974 to establish two experimental group homes in Monmouth, Oregon. Four children were placed in each home from either a state or private institution or from a family who could no longer maintain the child at home. The purpose of each home was to provide the residents with an environment to foster social skills and other behaviors that would allow them to return to their natural homes or foster homes in the local community (Gage, et al., 1977). Training programs were conducted in the group homes, coordination with the school was developed, and training programs were initiated with parents and/or significant people in the child's home environment. Either a house parent or shift-staff supervision was included within each group home. Similar resident gains were documented in each type of group home supervision.

Using an ecological analysis as a criterion of least restrictive alternative, the Teaching Research small group home model is an exemplary delivery system. A child with severe handicaps is removed from a physical environment of a large institution or unhealthy family situation and temporarily placed in a home with three other residents. An individual habilitation plan is formulated to match each individual's needs with appropriate intervention to enable him/her to return to a more normal, community environment. Once in the community, in-home services similar to those enumerated by Lensink are given to natural or foster parents. Thus, the small group home model for children is viewed as a temporary placement to remove children from a restrictive environment and prepare them to return to a more normal family setting.

Summary

As evidenced in the preceeding sections, many factors must be considered in deciding appropriate residences for persons with severe handicaps. In an attempt to attain the best possible living conditions for each individual, we must ask whether a continuum of services approach or a final stage support system approach is more appropriate for transitioning an individual to a least restrictive setting.

In a continuum of service model, sequenced options are available from which residents leave upon attaining proficiencies in community-based skills. For example, a resident may leave a state institution and reside in a large group home of twenty residents. Following a training phase at the home, a placement is made to a smaller home of five residents. Next, the resident may live in an apartment with a live-in companion and finally move into an apartment of his/her own with minimal support. An alternative approach would be to be place a resident from the institutional setting directly into his/her own apartment with a live-in companion. As the resident gains competencies in independent behavior, the live-in companion would gradually fade his/her assistance in a prescribed manner. Ohio has iterated the above concerns in a position paper prepared by the Community Services Subcommittee, Deinstitutionalization Task Force (1983). It is the Task Force Committees' contention that a final stage, home-centered approach is more advantageous for its citizens with severe handicaps. It is not the intent of this chapter to advocate strongly for either arrangement but to allow the reader to consider the merit of each based on the unique population to be served by your agency.

Chapter *3*

Evaluation of
Community-Living Options

W ITH THE continued decrease in federal dollars for social
services and an equal emphasis on a high degree of accountability for
the limited funds that are available, evaluation of residential options
for handicapped persons must become a high priority for members of
local, regional, and state planning agencies. A comprehensive
evaluation process developed for community-living options is
composed of three elements: needs assessment, formative evaluation,
and cost-effectiveness information. The purpose of a *needs assessment*
for community residential planners is to obtain a description of the
present state of affairs and provide documentation of a real need for
the initiation of a comprehensive residential plan for handicapped
individuals. *Formative evaluation* refers to the periodic assessment of
ongoing residential services in order to make decisions about whether
to continue the present delivery model or to develop alternative
residential options. Finally, a *cost-effectiveness analysis* refers to the
process of determining the "efficacy of a program in achieving given
goals measured substantively in relation to the program costs."
(Rossi, Freeman, & Wright, 1978, p. 242) The issues surrounding
needs assessment, formative evaluation and cost-effectiveness
analysis are now discussed in relation to the establishment of
community residential living options for individuals with severe
handicaps.

NEEDS ASSESSMENT

Bradley (1978) offers the following recommendation for the ingredients of a needs assessment:

1. A review of the current institutionalized population in state facilities whose home community is under the jurisdiction of the local agency to ascertain the level of functioning, income levels, age, and potential for movement into less restrictive living environments.
2. A survey of the community's handicapped persons residing in private institutional facilities to determine the appropriateness of ongoing placement and probable alternatives.
3. A review of persons on waiting lists for public and private facilities whose families reside in the agency's community to determine the characteristics of such persons and the possibility of alternatives to the services applied for.
4. Interviews with social and protective service workers to determine needs that they perceive among low income families with handicapped children.
5. A survey of private proprietary and nonprofit agencies serving handicapped persons to determine the provider assessment of need.
6. A canvass of other data sources including high-risk registers, school records, and vocational rehabilitation facilities (p. 65).

An additional component for a needs assessment is an evaluation of properties within a community that meet selected criteria for housing residents with severe handicaps.

When purchasing or constructing a home that will eventually become a residential facility, several features of this home should be considered. As family members approach the decision to buy a new home they usually consider three aspects of a home: beauty, enjoyment and growth. A new home should be pleasant to view, should provide space enough for recreation activities, both within the home and the surrounding property, and there should be features of the home that facilitates growth within its family members. These general thoughts concerning a new home are similar for those individuals involved in residential facility development.

The growth aspect of a residential facility is one that seeks features in the home that facilitates the learning of new skills by its residents. The residents of this home may never have experienced home-living experiences. Their new home should possess desirable features that allow the residents to practice behaviors that will help them to grow as individuals within the home and in their education, vocational and social endeavors. To accomplish this objective of securing a home that facilitates individual growth, each area of the home, outside and inside, should be analyzed for its appropriateness for each resident's growth. Programming for the residents should assist them in making progress in self-care, social, leisure time, vocational and other normalization skills. These skills can be learned in the home and the resident can make progress towards a more effective, normalized life style.

The following survey contains sample criteria that was developed to analyze specific areas of a home for optimal personal growth. The survey is not intended to be complete either in home areas covered or in criteria concerning each area, but is offered as a guide for obtaining this unique needs assessment information. Similar evaluations can be developed for both a new home or an existing facility. The most important consideration in conducting the survey is to perceive the home as a residence where individuals can grow mentally, physically, socially and emotionally.

MAJOR AREA: *Outside Environment (I)*
Topic: Proximity to Community Facilities (I-A)
                 Not Appropriate   See recommendations
*Definition: The area that is of close proximity to the home so that home members can readily benefit from the use of those facilities located in this area. (Judgment — a fifteen minute walk or drive would appear as close proximity.)

Criterion   **List**

• Recreational park(s) that can be used for
  active and/or quiet recreational activities:

• Playground(s) that can be used for active
  and/or quiet recreational activities:

• Recreational facilities that can be used for
  active and/or quiet recreational activities
  (e.g., YMCA, City Recreation Area...):

• Campgrounds that can be used for overnight
  camping:

• Store(s) that can be utilized for shopping
  purposes:

• Shopping center(s) that can be utilized for
  shopping purposes:

• Movie houses that are available:

- Specific entertainment centers that can be utilized (e.g., Art Museum, Ice Arena...):

- Churches in the area that are appropriate for ones spiritual life:

- Other (describe other criterion unique to this home):

*Create a list of these facilities; including a description of specific activities that can be participated in by home members at each site. Also, designate for those centers, where necessary, the fees required.

Diagram: (Draw map of surrounding area designating the different facilities that home members can use.)

Recommendations: (List recommendations for using the different facilities in the home's proximity area.)

(I-A)

Supplemental Sheet

Detailed List of Facilities in the Surrounding Area

Recreational Facilities:	Activities Available	Fee
(e.g., Smith Park — north on 1st street)	(softball, picnic area, swimming, play equipment)	50¢ swimming

Shopping Facilities:

Entertainment Facilities:

Churches:

MAJOR AREA: Outside Environment (I)
Topic: Garage(s) (I-B)
               Not appropriate   See recommendations

Definition: A sheltered place, that can be attached to the home, the major purpose for the storage of an automobile(s).

Criterion   **Comments**

- Area immediately surrounding the garage that can be used for active recreational purposes (e.g., basketball, shuffleboard...):

- Area inside the garage that can be utilized for a workshop setting (e.g., wood working, repair area...):

- Floor area inside the garage that can be used for active and/or quiet recreational activities:

- Rafters available where recreational equipment

may be hung (e.g., punching bag, swing...):

• Other (describe other criterion unique to this home):

Diagram: (Draw diagram of the garage giving dimensions.)

Recommendations: (List recommendation for using this garage area.)

MAJOR AREA: Outside Environment (I)
Topic: Driveway(s) (I-C)
                        Not appropriate   See recommendations

*Definition: That area of the property that serves as a pathway for vehicles entering from streets or alleyways.

(Recommend a roadblock when in use)

Criterion   **Comments**

• Driveway is of such dimension that it can be
  used for active recreational purposes
  (e.g., basketball, kickball...):

• Driveway can be utilized for quiet recreational
  activities (e.g., shuffleboard, hopscotch...):

• Driveway can be used for active play equipment
  when using safety precautions (e.g., tricycles,
  bicycles...):

• Driveway can be used for certain winter
  activities when using safety precautions
  (e.g., sledding, sliding...):

• Other (describe other criterion unique to this
  home):

Diagram: (Draw diagram of the driveway giving dimensions.)

Recommendations: (List recommendations for using the driveway area.)

*If more than one driveway, use separate sheets.

MAJOR AREA: Outside Environment (I)
Topic: Porch(es) (I-D)
                        Not appropriate   See recommendations

Definition: That covered outside area to the home that serves as an entrance and/or an open area adjunct to the walls of the house.

Criterion   **Comments**

• Area is of such a dimension that it can be
  used for small recreational activities
  (e.g., shuffleboard, ring toss...):

- Area is of a dimension that it can be used for small game activities (e.g., card games, checkers...):

- Area is of such a dimension and has safety precautions so that active play equipment can be used (e.g., tricycle, swing...):

- Area is of such a dimension that quiet activities can be pursued (e.g., reading, knitting...):

- Other (describe other criterion unique to this home.)

Diagram: (Draw diagram of porch area giving dimensions.)

Recommendations: (List recommendations for using this porch area.)

*If more than one porch area is present, use a separate sheet to describe each area.

MAJOR AREA: Home Environment (II)
Topic: Kitchen—Main Floor (II-A)
                   Not appropriate   See recommendations

*Definition:** That area of the home that is used for the preparation and the cooking of food.

Criterion   **Comments**

- Kitchen has adequate and safe facilities so that home members can cook food (stove, hot plate, frying pan, toaster...):

- Kitchen has adequate utensils so that home members can prepare meals and snacks (knives, spoons, cups, plan...):

- Kitchen has adequate cupboards and shelving so that home members can store food and kitchen supplies:

- Kitchen has adequate refrigeration space so that home members can adequately refrigerate food:

- Kitchen has adequate cleaning implements so that home members can adequately clean-up and maintain their kitchen:

- Other (describe other criterion unique to this home):

Diagram: (Draw diagram of the kitchen area giving dimensions.)

Recommendations: (List recommendations for using the kitchen area.)

*If more than one kitchen area, use separate sheet.

MAJOR AREA: Home Environment (II)

Topic: Living Room—Main Floor (II-B)
Not appropriate   See recommendations

Definition: That area that is on the main floor of the house that is used for social activities or the entertaining of guests. The room is usually filled with sofas, chairs, couch, etc.

Criterion   **Comments**

• Living room has a record player and records for home members use:

• Living room has adequate space for quiet leisure time activities (e.g., checkers, cards...):

• Living room has adequate shelving and storage space for books, newspapers, magazines...):

• Living room has adequate lighting for reading and close eye-hand leisure time activities (e.g., knitting, crocheting...):

• Living room has adequate space for small conversational groups:

• Living room has provisions for the care of small animals (e.g., aquarium, bird cage...):

• Living room has art objects that can be enjoyed by home members (e.g., paintings, pictures...):

• Living room has a television set that can be watched (television set *should be carefully* monitored):

• Other (describe other criterion unique to this home):

Diagram: (Draw diagram of the living room giving dimensions.)

Recommendations: (List recommendations for using the living room area.)

MAJOR AREA: Home Environment (II)

Topic: Dining Room (II-C)
Not appropriate   See recommendations

Definition: A room usually on the main floor of a home whose main purpose is for the consumption of meals.

Criterion   **Comments**

• Dining room has adequate space so that home

members can dine as a group.

* Dining room table is large enough so that home members can participate in quite leisure time activities (e.g., cards, puzzles...):

* Dining room is flexible enough so that active leisure time activities can be pursued (e.g., pool table, bumper pool table...):

* Dining room has adequate space for the storage of leisure time equipment (e.g., games, craft equipment...):

* Other (describes other criterion unique to this home):

Diagram: (Draw diagram of the dining room area giving dimensions.)

Recommendations: (List recommendations for using this dining room area.)

MAJOR AREA: Home Environment (II)

Topic: Recreational Room, Parlor (Additional room) (II-D)

Definition: Additional room(s) in the main floor area that can be used for different activities.

Criterion   **Comments**

* Area is of such a dimension that tables can be set up for quiet activities (e.g., table games, crafts...):

* Area is of such a dimension that active recreational activities can be pursued (e.g., pool, mat work tumbling...):

* Area can be used for the pursuit of craft activities (e.g. wood work, macrame...):

* Area can be used as a meeting area (e.g., group discussions...):

* Other (describe other criterion unique to home):

Diagram: (Draw a diagram of this area giving dimensions.)

Recommendations: (List recommendations for using this area.)

MAJOR AREA: Home Environment (II)

Topic: Bathroom(s) (II-F)
                    Not appropriate   See recommendations

Criteria   **Comments**

- Area has adequate space for instruction in bathing:

- Area has proper furnishing for instruction in showering:

- Area is appropriate for instruction in hair care:

- Area has adequate storage space for the instruction in how to keep hygienic possessions:

- Area has adequate mirrored space for self-monitoring of instructional progress:

- Area has adequate electrical outlet(s) for instruction in how to use electrical hygienic equipment (e.g., electric razor, hair dryer...):

- Other (describe other criterion unique to the home):

Diagram: (Draw diagram of the bathroom area(s) giving dimensions.)

Recommendations: (List recommendation for the bathroom area(s).)

MAJOR AREA: Home Environment (II)

Topic: Home Responsibilities (II-G)
Not appropriate   See recommendations

Criterion   **Comments**

- Chores and responsibilities are assigned in the kitchen area, and are posted, changed and supervised (e.g., dish washing, preparation of meals...):

- Chores and responsibilities are assigned in the living room and dining room areas, and are posted, changed, and supervised (e.g., vacuuming, setting table...):

- Chores and responsibilities are assigned in the bedroom and bathroom areas, and are posted, changed and supervised (e.g., making beds, cleans out bathtub...):

- Chores and responsibilities are assigned in other areas of the home and are posted, changed and supervised (e.g., recreational room, lab...):

• Other (describe other maintenance criterion unique to this home):

Maintenance Program: (Explain how the maintenance responsibilities of this home will be carried out—the assigning, posting, changing and supervising of these chores.)

Formative Evaluation

Once residential options have been established, there is a need to document the progress of each resident toward developing optimal functioning levels within the community. Such ongoing assessments can be obtained in many ways. In this section, assessment measures are roughly divided into qualitative and quantitative measurement procedures. Taylor and Bogdan (1981) describe qualitative evaluation as "inductive, holistic, and oriented to people's subjective experience." (p. 72) An observer uses an *inductive* approach when s/he enters a residential setting and only arrives at conclusions about the residents' functioning based on actual recorded data and not from previously written material about similar residents or similar environments. A *holistic* approach is an ecological interpretation of the resident's behavior considering the interrelationships among the individual resident's behaviors, the physical environment, the significant people involved with the welfare of the resident, and the prevailing norms, mores, and customs of the surrounding environment. Finally, qualitative evaluation is concerned with the *residents' observations* of what they are experiencing. The observer places a high value on this input as an important contribution for analyzing the satisfaction and feelings of each resident.

Quantitative evaluation procedures are characterized by the use of objective measurement procedures to pinpoint the resident's current functioning level. Adaptive behavior scales and criterion referenced assessment measures are examples of quantitative evaluation procedures that are described in this section. Adaptive behavior scales are measurement instruments designed to obtain general information about a resident's present functioning level. Criterion referenced assessments, however, are developed to measure a resident's progress on individual programs developed within each residential setting. Examples of qualitative and quantitative evaluation procedures are now described as they relate to formative evaluation.

Qualitative evaluation.

Edgerton and Langness (1978) advocate the use of participant-observation as a qualitative evaluation procedure to study the behavior of handicapped persons in community settings. In participant-observation, the observer's first objective should be to blend into the environment and become part of the resident's everyday interactions. This initial time-consuming adaptation phase will pay dividends later by allowing the observer to record narrative data for each resident in a nonreactive manner, thus, recording behavior as it would naturally occur. The participant-observer should be skilled at sequencing antecedent behavior, and consequence components of an observed event. By referring back to similar behavior episodes, the observer can pinpoint common events in the environment that were present before and after the behavior of interest. Multiple points of view of the same behavior by two or more observers can also increase the probability of pinpointing the key environmental influences of each resident's behavior. Thus, it is recommended that participant-observers initially work in teams and compare notes at the end of a recording session to assist each other in understanding the different events that occurred during the prior observation session. The longitudinal perspective obtained from the accumulation of recorded notes can also asisst the observer to look for common elements that impact each resident's behavior. Cyclic patterns can be documented that might be associated with such variables as visits from relatives, vacations, change of staff, work changes, and seasonal changes. An advantage of participant-observation as an evaluation technique is the ecological context in which events are viewed. A major question can be formulated: What are the relationships among the individual's behavior, co-residents' behavior, the physical structure of the residential facility, and the philosophy of the facility such as adherence to the principle of normalization?

In depth interviewing is a second qualitative measurement procedure for evaluating the daily functioning of deinstitutionalized individuals. Gollay, Freedman, Wyngaarden, and Kurtz (1978) described the community experiences of recently deinstitutionalized persons and purported to identify the critical factors related to their experiences. As part of their study, interviews were conducted with residents and significant people in the new living environment. Sample questions included:

Where would you rather live?
Would you rather live where you are now or at the institution?

What do you like about your work?
What do you not like about your work?

Similarly, Scheerenberger and Felsenthal (1977) interviewed seventy-five former residents of a public residential facility about their attitudes and comments on living in the community. Sample questions in their investigation included:

Can you go outside when you want to?
Can you hug someone if you want to?
Can you fix up (decorate) around your bed or your room?
Do you like the food here?

The responses from questions included in the Gollay et al., (1978) and Scheerenberger and Felsenthal (1977) interviews enable residential planners access to consumer satisfaction information. When residents are able to provide feedback about their perceptions and opinions, such information should be sought.

Participant-observation and in depth interviewing can be useful strategies to evaluate the progress of residents living in community settings. The interested reader is referred to Bogdan and Taylor (1975) for a more thorough discussion of these two qualitative evaluation procedures.

Quantitative evaluation.

It is common for residential licensing agencies to require an annual assessment to be conducted for each resident. The purpose of this assessment is to obtain a general description of each resident's progress over time. Usually the assessment instrument is an adaptive behavior scale similar to the AAMD Adaptive Behavior Scale (Nihira, Foster, Shellhaas, & Leland, 1974), the Minnesota Developmental Programming System (Bock &Weatherman, 1976), or the Progress Assessment Chart (Gunzburg, 1974). The information gathered from these instruments may be useful to generally describe an individual's functioning level in relation to other similar individuals on the items of the scale. For example, the Minnesota Developmental Programming System contains twenty statements in eighteen domains requiring a response of either always, more than half the time, less than half the time, or never. A sample statement from the Recreation, Leisure Time domain is "initiates self-involvement in a hobby not including reading or watching TV." An evaluator can obtain a general impression of the level of functioning an individual is presently at but not how well that resident has performed on an individual hobby or recreation activity. For this reason criterion referenced evaluation procedures are recommended.

In the context of this chapter criterion referenced evaluations refer to measures of the progress of individuals on specific tasks. The purpose of criterion referenced assessment is not to gain a global picture of an individual's functioning level but to assess the present skill deficit on a task and evaluate the progress during an intervention program. A task is divided into its component steps and these steps are then sequenced in a logical order. This specific criterion referenced evaluation is called task analytic assessment. Usually the criterion is established by observing how chronological-age peers perform the task and take into account any adaptations that are needed for the handicapped resident.

Cost-Effectiveness

The task of evaluating residential options on a cost-effectiveness basis is difficult. In public residential facilities careful records are kept to document the expenditure of monies from external funding sources. However, in smaller facilities such detailed record keeping is seldom observed, especially in foster home and semiapartment placements. Another reason for this difficulty relates to the factors included in determining the costs and benefits for each facility. Specifically, are societal costs included in the cost-effective analysis? Gross (1977) describes societal costs as "the dollar we spend today...not just a simple dollar, but must also be looked at in terms of the foregone opportunity of spending the money in other ways." (p. 428) Other factors pertinent to any comparison of cost-effectiveness is determining the dollar figure attributed to volunteer persons, donated items, practicum site for students, involvement in research, etc. When Yates (1977) tried comparing his residential program with other local programs he found the other programs lacked the pertinent ingredients for such a comparison. Yates's dilemma represents the rule rather than the exception found in cost-effectiveness comparisons.

Given the above global limitations, all of the studies comparing institutions and community living alternatives reviewed by Heal and Laidlaw (1980) contained evidence that it was less expensive to place developmentally disabled individuals into the community, especially into natural or foster homes. National studies by Baker, Seltzer, and Seltzer (1977), Conley (1973), and Scheerenberger (1978) as well as regional comparisons by Gardner (1977) in Ohio, Heal and Daniels (1978) in Wisconsin, Intagliata, WIller, and Cooley (1979) in New

York, Jones and Jones (1976) in Massachusetts, and Peat, Marwick, Mitchell, & Company (1977) in Illinois were included in the Heal and Laidlaw (1980) analysis.

Two additional studies; not included in the Heal and Laidlaw (1980) analysis, contain evidence that the difference between institutional and community facility placement may not be as great as some of the earlier studies had indicated. Howse (1980) describes the average institutional costs in 1977 for New York City to be $29,000.00. As a comparison, the range of costs for community residential placement was from $8,000.00 to $35,000.00. Howse still maintains that "on the balance, the community program is less expensive than institutionalization and offers a higher quality of service." (p. 71) Gage, Fredericks, Baldwin, Moore, and Grove (1977) compared the monthly costs of three alternative placements for children in Oregon and found that the state institution for developmentally disabled to be $918.00 per child, a manager model group home to be $902.34 per child and a parent model group home to be $998.81 per child.

As accountability systems and cost documentation become more sophisticated (a comprehensive example is outlined by Heal and Laidlaw), comparisons between institutional and community residential placements may be more valid. As a word of caution, Howse (1980) emphasizes that "the initial arguments for developing community programs must be service and rights based and not just cost based, because it takes time to realize cost savings in a deinstitutionalization program." (p. 71) Thus, even though initial costs for residential options may be higher than an institutional environment, residents have a greater probability of gaining skills that will lessen the amount of money needed in the future for their direct support.

Summary

Included in this chapter were recommendations for the evaluation of community-living options for persons with severe handicaps. Needs assessment, formative evaluation and cost-effectiveness analysis are the three critical areas that were described in the previous sections. Information from these three areas contribute to the services that will become more critical as accountability demands increase. An efficiently operated residence must have well formulated action plans in each of these three evaluation areas.

Chapter 4

Financing a Residential Home

Major challenges face administrators of residential homes for individuals with severe handicaps in the area of fiscal management. Every aspect of the residential facility is dependent upon adequate financial support, from the expense of providing nutritional breakfasts, to taking the residents to a basketball game or purchasing summer clothing. It all costs money. And the money necessary to meet residential facility costs has not always been readily obtainable or adequate to meet the spiraling expenses of maintaining an efficient home environment for each resident.

The reality of many financial difficulties facing the operation of a residential home is crisis budgetary management; maintaining enough financial support to meet basic operational needs but not necessarily a minimal financial crisis situation. For example, there is a continual need to anticipate expenditures like major repairs on the residential van or the purchasing of new fire detection equipment for the facility. Too often residential facility budgets can only handle additional facility costs by securing the money from other budget lines, such as therapeutic, recreational or clothing funds. This type of crisis management budgeting only hinders the residential facility's ability to best serve its residents.

What is needed, therefore, for residential facilities to overcome such financial problems is that the residential facility strives diligently towards securing a solid financial base. This includes a funding base that allows the residential facility to provide the most adequate residential care and programming and at the same time allows for a cash flow to meet other reasonable emergencies.

This chapter will assist individuals concerned with the administering of the financial aspects of a residential facility. It begins with a discussion of the different financial options available to residential facilities and concludes with a consideration of financial strategies that will assist in the budgetary management of the residential facility.

Financial Support Options

There are a variety of options available in obtaining financial support for a residential facility. A single financial option or a combination of options can be used. Each financial approach has a positive as well as a negative aspect to its particular support base. Administrators within residential facilities will need to evaluate each financial consideration and determine the most efficient method in handling their own particular budgetary concerns.

Private Funding

Financial support of a residential facility can be secured from private sources. Private funding receives its name because its funding base is not connected with any local, state or federal general revenue—money received from taxation. The funds are secured from individuals or special groups that are a part of the private sector of the community.

Individuals who are willing to financially support a residential home include a broad spectrum of sources within the community. Financial support of a residential facility by an individual, although not common, has been observed and residential facilities have been partially or fully supported by this benefactor approach. The reason for contributions varies from individual to individual. However, the most common reasons would be a concern for individuals with handicaps, often a family member, or a desire to contribute something meaningful for society.

Special groups within a community are willing to support or assist in the financial endeavors of a residential home. The most common are church organizations. Church supported residential facilities have been established throughout the country. Almost all church denominations have been represented in some type of residential commitment. A church's willingness to undertake such a venture is in many ways similar to the willingness of an individual to offer his or her assistance. A concern exists to help the residents and is often championed by a parent or parents in the church organization who have a child with a handicap, or a desire to contribute financially to a very meaningful and worthwhile cause.

Church organizations are not the only special groups in the community willing to finance residential homes. Service groups have been involved in many instances in residential financing. However, service group monies are usually donated for specific purposes. An example of special purpose funding would be the local Optimist Club's purchase of a specially equipped van for transporting residents with physical handicaps. There has been a recent trend for the business and industrial community to become involved in the private funding of special residential projects. Near several medical centers, the national McDonald's Corporation is involved in transient homes for parents and family members of seriously ill children so that families may stay close to hospitalized children.

Advantages

No matter what source of private funding may be available, there are real advantages to this type of financing of residential homes. Private funding usually permits budgetary decisions to be made by the administration of the residential facility, recognizing them as the experts in providing a specialized service. Service group support also has an advantage in addition to monetary contributions. Service group members who have a special talent or skill such as an electrician, plumber or an accountant can assist the home by donating their skills to the facility. Finally, private funds may not be so rigidly tied to specific budget items, as in other funding options, so that budgeting can be more fluidly adjusted.

Disadvantages

Private funding, however, has some disadvantages. Foremost, a longitudinal funding commitment to the residential facility may not be apparent. It would be poor planning to base the future of the home on the spurious commitment from one private source. Additionally, there is the possibility that the private funding source may be or may become philosophically opposed to the daily operations of the administrators of the facility. Such differences can often be detrimental to the facility. Finally, private funding, even though it may be longitudinally committed, may have difficulty in keeping up with rising inflation in the economy. The funding source may be so tightly committed that any increases in operational costs would be beyond the ability of the fund to provide adequate assistance.

In summary, some residential facilities are being funded by private community sources. Private funds in support of residential financing has its primary advantage when the management of the facility can operate in an autonomous manner. However, long-range residential commitment by the private funding source can be a real serious disadvantage. Care must be exercised in relying too heavily on this funding base.

Private Funding

Advantages:
- management autonomy
- services beside monetary benefits
- budget flexibility

Disadvantages:
- lack of longitudinal monetary commitment
- philosophical differences
- inflational problems

Profit Funding

Profit funding for residential homes is in evidence in many communities. Common with private funding, this funding source originates from either an individual or a special group of individuals willing to invest in a business proposition. However, profit funding differs from private funding when these funds are generated on the premise that the contributors can earn a profit from their monetary venture. Financial backing of the residential facility from these investors who desire some form of monetary profit, makes this type of residential home a business.

Investing for profit in the operation of a residential home has been a common model in the financing of nursing care facilities for the aged. The investor can realize a profit from an investment in different ways, including:

a) straight profit after expenses and taxation
b) tax sheltering of a percentage of the investor's income
c) tax allowance for an apportion of the income
d) capital gains after a period of time
e) eventual sale of a portion or all of the business

The business aspect of profit funding support for residential facilities can be organized in several ways. The most common method has been to form a board of directors comprised of the individuals who have invested their money in the facility. When a board of directors hires an administrator to operate the residential facility, the administrator is responsible for the total operation of the facility and undertakes the responsibility to make a profit for the investors. Administrators who operate within this model generally report on a regular basis to the board of directors concerning the operation of the facility.

A different organizational model from the active board of directors model is where the investor(s) operate as silent partners. This type of organizational structure occurs when the investors function in a much less formal manner than as members of a board of directors. The investors would remain silent as long as the residential facility is earning an equitable profit on their investment. Although not a common organizational model, it usually involves a limited number of investors.

Advantages

There are a number of advantages to the profit funding of residential facilities for persons with varying degrees of handicapping conditions. One of the principal advantages is that the investors have a solid financial base from which to finance the residential facility. The source of funding support for the facility may be given enough flexibility to reduce the bureaucracy common to other types of funding sources. Additionally, the expertise of the investors can be a real strength to the facility in the area of budgeting and fund raising. Knowledgeable business persons can create a very solvent residential facility with a potential for an extremely efficient and effective residential setting.

Disadvantages

The major disadvantages of this funding base can be quickly stated in the two words: profit motive. Investors might only be interested in making money from the facility and could do a great deal of harm to the humanitarian aspects of the facility. *Profit blindness* could seriously affect all phases of the residential operation, from programming to general health needs of the residents.

When considering profit financing for a residential facility, special care must be taken so that profit motivation is appropriately balanced with resident care. When appropriate resident care is provided, a profit-minded group of investors can operate an efficient and effective residential facility with definite advantages for the facility.

Profit Funding

Advantages:
- solid financial base
- management flexibility
- financial expertise of the investors

Disadvantage:
- extreme profit motivation

Local Agency Funding

In recent years, local agencies concerned with individuals with severe handicaps have become more involved with the development and funding of residential facilities. A county board of mental retardation is an example of a local agency that may become involved in providing residential services for individuals within their geographic area. These local agencies have begun to provide this service because they feel a responsibility to offer appropriate, normalized living experiences that coexist with educational, vocational and social aspects in the life of individuals with severe handicaps.

When a local agency makes the decision to develop and finance local residential facilities for its citizens, it must seek local funding sources for its establishment. Though local funds can be secured in different ways, the most common method is through a local tax levy. A levy is presented to the community on a ballot and is a request for a certain taxable contribution from the community. The approval of a levy by the community provides the local agency with the funding base for the support of the residential facility, although possible state, federal and private funds may also be involved.

Usually, when community support has been provided, the local agency establishes an advisory board to assist in the operation of the facility. Advisory board members appoint an administrator of the facility to provide the daily expertise necessary for the effective operation of the facility. The advisory board selects an administrator who is in tune with the local agency's philosophical and pragmatic concerns for the operation of the residential facility. It is important that the facility's administration and the advisory board establish a cooperative working relationship. When this occurs, the advisory board's policy is followed through in a positive manner within the facility. A conflict between the administration of the facility and the advisory board will likely have a detrimental effect upon the facility's operations.

Advantages

An advantage of local agency funding occurs when the administration of the residential facility remains a part of a local advocacy group. If the local agency has the knowledge and understanding of appropriate residential management, local administrators who are advocates of residential programming can be a real advantage. Another advantage to this funding source is that community individuals who are handicapped may be best served by a local residential facility that is knowledgeable of their particular needs. Community pride also may be an advantage in that the community is proud of what it can accomplish for its citizens who are handicapped.

Disadvantages

Disadvantages to local agency funding are generally the opposite of the advantages. If the local agency is a mediocre advocate for handicapped populations and also has little understanding of the objectives of an effective residential facility, local control will likely be detrimental. Also, the placement of residents into a residential facility may, if not closely monitored, become a form of favoritism for some individuals. In such instances, the selection of residential placements have little to do with the specific needs of a client. Community pride can also turn into community hostility if the facility is forced upon the community or if the management of the facility is perceived as inadequate by the community. For example, if neighbors believe that the residential facility's staff is unable to control residents' behavioral problems, the local community will certainly have serious doubts about the facility's ability to maintain its operation. Reactions may take the form of letters to the editor of the local newspaper or petitions to local funding agencies.

In summary, a local agency's development and funding of residential facilities has reached quite an impetus during recent years.

48   *A User's Guide*

The major advantage for this funding source is that local concern can generate a community willingness to provide residential service to the community's residents who are handicapped. Discretion, however, must be used in the local agency's management of the facility so that appropriate selection of the residents is guaranteed and that healthy community relations are established and maintained.

Local Agency Funding

Advantages
  • local control of the residential facility
  • selection of residents from the local community
  • community pride in local accomplishment
Disadvantages:
  • local agency's inability to manage residential facilities
  • selection of residents based on the wrong reasons
  • establishment of poor community relations

Purchase of Service (State Funding)

Purchase of service funding refers to funds that are usually received from state government agencies for a specified type of care. State governments, in providing purchase of service funding, provide monetary reimbursements to local community facilities for specific services rendered to the residents. State purchase of service monies is the most prevalent form of residential funding pattern found throughout the United States.

There are several reasons why purchase of service funding patterns have become a common source of residential financial support. Prevalent among these reasons is that state institutions for the handicapped throughout the country have made a commitment to depopulate the number of residents within their facility. This impetus of deinstitutionalization to decrease the number of residents within institutions has led to the alternative placement of such institutionalized individuals to local community facilities. Rather than reimbursing state institutions for the care of its residents, state government agencies have willingly supported the least restrictive alternative of residential facility placement. State officials' sensitivity to the criticism of the institutional model and the realization in many instances of lower funding expenditures to the smaller residential facilities have encouraged the development of such homes.

The stimulation of local community interest and support for residential facilities has been an additional reason for state government support of local facilities. In many communities, residential projects have not become operative. By providing funding incentives for residential facilities throughout the state, local communities are becoming aware of the benefits of placement within their own community.

Purchase of service funding can be obtained and monitored in many ways. State governments have organized respective agencies into regional or district offices, making communication with the local communities easier to establish. Also, regional organizations create a closer contact with community resource personnel within each designated region or district. Within a regional concept of state organization, funding for residential facilities is contracted through the district office (i.e., a regional Office of Mental Retardation). The contracting for services rendered and the monitoring of this contract would occur through the district office, although final approval of the contracted residential facilities occurs at the state level.

Another arrangement for purchase of service funding is when the state government has one central state office for the handicapped. This central state office is located with other state agencies in the state capital. Instead of state government involvement at a more local level, state funding for residential facilities are contracted through the central office. Under this arrangement, the state agency responsible for purchase of service monies will have total responsibility for all contracted residential facilities throughout the state.

In the State of Ohio, a contractual agreement for the operations of residential facilities for individuals with mental retardation and developmental disabilities (MR-DD) is written into agreements with county boards of MR-DD. The county boards have been given the responsibility by law to provide a comprehensive service plan, which is reviewed annually and revised as needed. The law specifies that the plan should include:

5123:2-1-02 Administration
(ii) The number or residential placements to be developed or eliminated in the county, the characteristics of those individuals for whom the placements are needed, the type of facilities to be developed (i.e., Family Homes, Group Homes, Specialized Care and Independent Living), the anticipated sources of funding such facilities and the anticipated sources of funds to support such facilities.

Once a county board's comprehensive service plan has been developed and approved, a request is made for purchase of service monies. When submitting their plans, county boards should be able to provide proof that all other sources of residential funding have been considered and that these other sources are not available. These records of revenue searching help protect the state from providing purchase of service money from its general fund when other sources of funding revenue could be secured by the county boards.

Advantages

A first advantage is that the state government may have a more realistic understanding of the cost of financing the operation of a residential home than do individual community members. State agency representatives are involved in long-range residential operations and have knowledge of the expense of various residential options. Their calculation of per diem (cost per day, per resident) may be more in line with actual cost. In many instances, the state agency will have a broader base of information concerning residential home operation than local organizations because of their statewide frame of reference in being involved in similar endeavors. There is also the possibility in states that have regional offices that more consistent monitoring of residential facilities will occur.

Disadvantages

The most apparent disadvantages of dealing with any state agency is size and learning to cope with the bureaucracy inherent in state government and state personnel who may have too little or too much responsibility towards state residential facilities. The problem for many community residential facilities is learning to wade through numbers of state personnel in finding assistance from the right person. At times, such efforts by community residential facilities can be extremely frustrating. Another disadvantage to such purchase of service funding is the inherent vulnerability of state funds to internal and external economic conditions of the state and country. State allocations of funds for state projects can have good and bad years — recently, state funding has experienced a lean support base.

Purchase of service funding through state government involvement is the most common type of financial support of residential facilities throughout the country. State organizational structures for handling residential funding come from either regional or central offices. Purchase of service funding has its advantages. However, one must be aware of the bureaucracy in dealing with state governments.

Purchase of Service Funding
Advantages:
- appropriate funding allocations
- broader base knowledge of residential facilities
- more consistent monitoring

Disadvantages:
- bureaucracy
- vulnerability of funds to economic conditions

Medicaid: Title XIX (Federal Funding)

Medicaid has been a federal funding source that has been received by state and local agencies concerned with residential facilities. Medicaid is a federal assistance program that pays medical bills for eligible individuals. Although labeled as a total federal program similar to Medicare, Medicaid is really a federal-state partnership, a partnership whereby each state designs its own Medicaid program within federal guidelines.

Though eligibility criteria vary somewhat from state to state, Medicaid is basically for groups of needy and low income individuals that include:

a) the aged (over 65 years)
b) the blind
c) the disabled
d) members of families with dependent children
e) other special needs children

Residential facilities for persons with handicaps become eligible for federal-state funding because they often have individuals within their facility who meet eligibility requirements. Specialized residential facilities serving residents who are Medicaid eligible enable that residential facility to apply for total facility funding. Thus, a residential facility having met stringent Medicaid requirements can receive Medicaid funding for the operation of the facility. The Medicaid total facility requirements are quite comprehensive in their coverage of eligibility criteria. The requirements are usually organized into a number of broad categorical headings that are further defined into more specific headings and then detailed into a carefully written requirement. Sample criteria include:

Administrative Policies and Procedures

Philosophy, objectives, and goals

The facility must have written policies and procedures that insure the civil rights of all residents.

Training and Habilitation Services

Required Services
    The facility must provide training and habilitation services to all residents, regardless of age, degree of retardation, or accompanying disabilities or handicaps.

Example of Broad Categorical Headings

Admission and Release
Personnel Policies
Resident Living
Dental Service
Food and Nutrition Services
Medical Services
Recreational Service
Records

In order to obtain Medicaid certification, procedures must be initiated by the residential facility and finalized by a Medicaid report. A formal letter of application is sent to the appropriate state Medicaid office. A fee is included in filing this application. Before the application is filed, careful consideration should be given to the reasonableness of obtaining the certification. To reach this decision, a residential facility should conscientiously study each standard in relationship to its own facility. If a decision is made to apply, the application is filed and a Medicaid survey team begins a series of visits. These survey teams evaluate the facility against its published standards. Finally, a written report is issued from the Medicaid office and contains a statement of acceptability or unacceptability of the facility for Medicaid funding.

Advantages

The main advantage to federal-state funding is assurance of adequate funding. Medicaid funding has been at a per diem rate that has established a solid financial base for residential facilities receiving funds. Also, a residential facility that meets comprehensive standards has the ability to provide adequate service to its residents. Finally, the solid financial base of Medicaid funding often provides for adequate auxiliary staff who can provide the appropriate services that are required in the comprehensive Medicaid standards.

Disadvantages

This type of funding, as with any governmental intervention or bureaucracy, is itself a disadvantage. In the case of Medicaid funding, bureaucracy means personnel responsible for recording, gathering and filing of paperwork. Additionally, the concept of normalization as it relates to a residential home becomes a questionable objective because of some Medicaid regulations. Governmental regulations often appear as a rigid confrontation to a normalized home environment. Certain Medicaid regulations reflect more of a medical-institutional environment than a normalized residential environment and thus constitutes a definite disadvantage. Federal legislation is pending to address many of the deficits in the Medicaid formula for funding community residential facilities.

Medicaid funding has become a prominent source for larger residential facilities. While there are definite advantages to this funding base, not all facilities should seek these funds. Residential facilities may seriously inhibit a normalized life style for its residents by having to follow stringent Medicaid regulations. Careful scrutiny of the Medicaid regulations must be made by those responsible for deciding on this funding source before a formal application is processed.

Federal Funding: Medicaid

Advantages:
- solid financial base
- appropriate resident service
- appropriate auxiliary staff

Disadvantages:
- bureaucracy
- difficulty in providing normalized living environment

In summary, the preceding sections contained a brief review of several financial support options available to residential facilities. Planning members of a residential facility must carefully evaluate all financial options that are possible for the facility to have a solid financial base to reach its potential in providing an adequate normalized life style for its residents.

Other Financial Considerations

The following financial considerations are offered as suggestions in handling regular budgetary matters rather than the broader based financial support of the facility that was previously discussed. These budgetary matters can assist the facility to function in a proficient manner.

Establish a reserve fund

If the residential budget has any monetary reserve possibility, establish a separate fund for this reserve. This advice is especially sound for those facilities operating with state funding. State funds are usually based on a biennial budget and the second year of this budget can be a reduction year. This reduction in the residential budget is quite possible when the state government is spending money over its projected time table and state revenues are less than predicted. This reserve fund can help the facility get through unexpected reduction periods. It is also sound business practice, even when not receiving state funds to anticipate emergency situations. At the beginning of any fiscal year there is a strong tendency to spend monies much more readily. The annual budget apears large and seemingly its dollars will last forever. It is much more prudent, however, to spend the residential dollars in a wise manner and at the same time build a reserve towards some possible monetary crisis situation.

Purchase residential items with a budget in mind

There is a real savings to residential facilities that purchase facility items with the scrutiny of a seasoned shopper. Savings can be realized by purchasing items in large quantities. Also, those in charge of purchasing must carefully observe the savings announced in newspapers, shopping guides and other such advertisements. Additional savings can occur with special arrangements with businesses in the community for discounts because of a consistent purchasing of items at their stores. Friends of the residential facility can also collect food and discount coupons to assist in further savings.

Protect overtime pay

Administrators who are responsible for issuing paychecks should closely monitor overtime payments. Employees who are regularly drawing time and a half pay are draining the personnel budget. If the personnel budget is being depleted at too fast a rate because of administrative/employee abuse of the overtime payment, adjustments must be implemented. Nothing can deplete the funds of a residential facility more quickly than a lackadaisical policy concerning overtime pay. For example, if a residential employee is earning a base pay of five dollars an hour, this same worker at time and a half will receive seven dollars and fifty cents an hour for basically the same work. If such a situation becomes quite commonplace and many employees receive time and a half pay, the facility has quickly increased its pay scale to the point where the facility is spending a much greater amount on staff wages than originally allocated in the budget. Such payment practices will rapidly deplete a facility's budget.

Utilize voluntary community resources to save funds

As will be discussed in chapter six on the utilization of volunteers, a residential facility has a valuable resource potential available in the use of volunteers. These individuals are identified as willing community members who bring many diverse skills and talents to the facility. Many of these individual skills reduce facility expenses. Each volunteer worker who assists the residential facility is saving money for the facility. If the administration of the facility had to hire additional personnel, even at minimum wage, the savings realized by volunteer staff can amount to a nice savings.

Explore energy conservation

Most residential facilities have high cost in the area of utilities. A residential facility that has many individuals in and out of the facility throughout the day and night is not an average family dwelling in the consumption of electrical, gas, oil, water and other utility considerations. Heavy use of the facility's utilities and rising utility costs are an ongoing drain upon facility funds. Administrators of residential facilities must reduce costs by practical conservation. They should seek advice in energy conservation by consulting experts.

Summary

It is apparent that there are a number of options available for residential funding. The funding options detailed in this chapter are not usually used as single sources of financing. Most residential facilities have a combination of funding sources. The critical issue in funding, however, is not which funding source is used, but how stable such a funding base is over the years. In addition to securing a sound funding base, careful scrutiny of daily budgetary matters should be undertaken so that savings can be realized by the facility.

Chapter 5

Transitioning Residents from Previous Living Environments

Just about everyone in this highly transient world has moved to a new home. The experience of moving leaves one with a feeling of ambivalence, feelings of joy-sadness, hope-dejection and excitement-indifference. We desire the new, but cling to the old. The new home is exciting, but the old residence was comfortable. These emotions accompany most individuals when they are uprooted from one home to another. Many individuals with severe handicaps are not afforded the opportunity to select a new residence. This decision is often in the hands of institutional personnel, client managers, advocates and/or parents or guardians. The decision to transfer a resident is not malevolently decided, but in almost all instances is sought for the good of the individual. Such secondhand decisions, however, do not ease the emotional upheaval of a move for the resident. In most instances, this decision only serves to magnify the displaced individual's feelings of ambivalence.

One might argue that given the physical, emotional and mental conditions of individuals with severe handicaps such concerns are not relevant. The priority to move the individual to a new residence is the utmost concern. The emotions of the residents seem to be a distant second. This ordering of priorities is a denial of basic human rights, to choose where one will live.

Concerned residential personnel must carefully develop a displacement strategy that will provide the resident with an enriched home environment while overcoming the displacement blues. This chapter contains suggestions on ways to reduce this problem. Each residential facility, however, has its own uniqueness and must foster its own manageable solutions. No matter what solution is formulated to solve this displacement problem, a priority should be a genuine concern for the resident's well being. If human concern comes first, reasonable solutions will soon follow.

Gradual Introduction to the Home

Displaced residents arrive at a new home from a variety of previous living environments including family homes, foster homes, state and private institutions. The new residents bring with them experiences from previous dwellings. Beyond professional beliefs that the new dwelling is a more adequate home, residents should experience warmth and attachment to their new home. For the residents to perceive this warmth in their new home, they must be gradually introduced to these new surroundings. Granted, there are emergency situations that dictate a rapid movement of individuals to new residential settings, however, such situations should be minimized. Individual residential movement will best be accomplished when careful planning of the move is undertaken.

Gradual movement of residents from one facility to another will allow residential personnel time to work with each resident. This preparation time can be used to prepare the new resident emotionally and mentally for a change (often drastic) in their life style. If a gradual movement is possible, the following suggestions should be considered:

a **Include the individual in the decision process.** Whenever possible, the individual, even with only minimum capabilities, should be part of the displacement decision. This suggestion is too often disregarded when a residential move reaches determination.

b **Inform the individual as quickly as possible.** When the individual was not a part of the decision to move to a new residence, s/he needs to know as soon as possible that a decision has been reached. Capabilities of the resident will dictate the method and technique of relaying this message. Such capabilities will also control the individual's understanding of the decision.

c **Contact all individuals who have a guardian-like role with the resident.** Advocates and guardians can assist in creating a smooth residential transition.

d   **Describe to the resident what the new home will be like.** Familiarity with a new dwelling can soothe initial anxieties. Residential discussions, for those individuals who can benefit from these conversations, are quite meaningful. The use of pictures from the new home can also be beneficial when informing the individual of the new living environment.

e   **A visit to the present facility by individuals who are a part of the new residence should be arranged.** A visit will initiate the breaking down of barriers of unfamiliarity. Understandings and friendships can begin to flourish. This visit could include an administrative representative, a residential care worker, facility programmer and residents of the new facility.

f   **A visit, or a sequence of visits, should be arranged to the new residence.** A visit to the residence can acclimate the person to eventual surroundings. When possible, these visits should be for an extended time period with an accompanying advocate from the present facility. Even though these visits can be time-consuming and expensive, the positive benefits to the resident can be well worth the expense.

g   **Enable the new resident to join in group activities that are a part of the new home.** The new resident should be included in the home activities of the new dwelling. A special leisure time activity (movie, basketball game, dance or similar events) would be a good introduction for the new resident. Caution, however, should be exercised so that the resident does not become anxious by immediate demands and unfamiliar experiences.

A major priority in transitioning residents from one facility to another is to proceed gradually. Planning for a gradual move allows for a higher probability that a pleasant personal adjustment by the resident will occur.

Preserving Some of the Old

Too often, the new resident has been moved to a living environment with nothing more than a suitcase or bag filled with clothes. Any possessions sometimes do not follow the resident. This failure to preserve aspects of the old residence only serves to make the move more difficult.

An effort on the part of persons involved in moving the individual should be concerned with transferring familiar items from the previous residence. If the resident is capable of choosing objects to bring along, obviously this should be granted. When an individual decision is not possible, obtain input from other individuals who are familiar with the resident. Ask those friends to list the things that the resident possessed in the previous setting that should continue to be owned in the new residence. Property rights of the resident must be respected. When these rights become an issue, understandings must be reached to either replace the items at the previous residence or duplicate them at the new home. Appropriate judgements with the following considerations will assist in making some decisions:

a   **Pictures/paintings/posters:** visual objects that the resident has enjoyed should be moved to the new residence.
b   **Bedding:** blankets and/or pillows that have been a part of the individual's bedding should be moved.
c   **Simple furniture:** inexpensive furniture items such as a pipe rack or a tie/belt rack will help bring some of the old into the new residence.
d   **Personal items:** items which the individual has used on a regular basis such as a coffee mug or ash tray should be included.
e   **Leisure time items:** basic games, books, magazines or craft items that the resident has enjoyed should be transported.

The previous list is only a sample of the many items that could be moved to the new home. Too often, residents have been transported to new living environments but not really moved. Move the resident's personal items to help foster a warm and pleasant transition.

Personalizing the New Home

The new resident should be readily assimilated into the new home. This feeling of belonging can occur most quickly when the resident understands what part of the home is now his/her personal area. An understanding should be reached so that the resident comprehends that basic rights and privacy exist for all home members. Take time to assist the new resident in the comprehension of new personal property. Personalization of space and property is an important understanding to reach for the new resident. Every effort should be made to help the new resident feel that not only will s/he be living in this home but that the property has become a part of their possessions.

Quickly establish personal items for the resident including a bedspread, bureau, bed table, toiletry items, clothes hamper, wall pictures, and craft items. A word of caution: placing personal identification on each individualized item in the home can create an institutional atmosphere. Identification of personalized items is important for the protection of personal property but other systems can be used. A log book, for example, recording each resident's property, with accurate descriptive identification, would suffice. This system would eliminate the need for always having to tag items throughout the home. Identification tags on household items are not homelike.

Transferring Relevant Information

Each resident should have a file of relevant information that is transferred to his new home. This information is critical to the welfare of the resident. Medical information would be at the top of the list of necessary information. Included in this category are medications, allergies, and history of seizure activity. This medical information should be supplied to the new home in advance of the resident's arrival. When this information arrives with the resident, there is not enough lead time to digest the material. Appropriate measures can be established to insure the resident's health and safety when these records are made available prior to the resident's arrival.

An additional consideration related to medical information is obtaining information on who to contact concerning unique medical conditions. Upon reviewing the resident's medical records, questions may surface about the resident's present physical condition. For example, questions on present medications, seriousness of high blood pressure, possible food allergies and special diets that have been recommended are important considerations. Contact must be made with individuals who have knowledge of the necessary information: parents, guardians, physicians and nurses. If addresses and phone numbers of these individuals are not provided in the medical records, immediate acquisition of this information must occur.

An individual who has previous knowledge of the resident should carefully interpret sensitive medical information to the staff members of the new residence. This conference should precede the arrival of the new resident and give all individuals an opportunity to ask questions and acquire important information. Too little knowledge of the new resident can create serious problems and adjustment difficulties. These problems can be avoided if appropriate communication channels are in operation.

Resident records also need to be kept in a secure but readily available filing cabinet. This file system will protect the resident's privacy rights and be sure that only authorized personnel have access to these records. Relevant resident information is an important ingredient in assisting the new resident in adjusting to a new facility. Important questions need to be addressed. The following list contains a sample of necessary documents:

a **Medical:** important current medical information must be documented, highlighting serious medical problems and if appropriate, detailed reports concerning medications.
b **Social history:** an extensive background report elaborating salient events in the resident's life.
c **Psychological report:** a description of the emotional stability of the individual and highlights of specific behavior problems.
d **Special physical-sensory-neurological report:** when necessary a report dealing with special conditions or deprivations concerning the resident should be included.
e **Intellectual functioning:** this information should reflect the intellectual maturity of the individual in relationship to problem solving, everyday judgement, generalization, communication and how it influences the daily progress of the resident.
f **Adaptive behavior:** knowledge of how the new resident handles daily living skills such as eating, toileting, bathing, etc. Suggestive comments on how to handle problem areas with these skills should be delineated.
g **Special techniques and methods:** information that gives prominence to special handling of the resident when specific problems exist, including strategies that have worked in the past such as specific behavior modification techniques.

Establishing Personal Relationships

An individual entering a new home and a new community will need to establish some personal relationships early in this experience. Isolation and loneliness can be quickly felt by the new resident unless appropriate procedures are undertaken that are sensitive to the individual's need for establishing meaningful relationships with others. Each resident will vary in the number and degree of such relationships, but all will need some type of contact. Guidelines for establishing personal interactions should provide avenues for residents to establish appropriate personal contacts early in their new home experience. Assigning a staff advocate for the new resident early in the placement process is a beginning step. This staff member will be resonsible for assisting the new resident to satisfactorily adjust to the new home. Even before the individual arrives at the new residence, a staff advocate should be involved in meeting the resident, reviewing records and participating in plans for the resident's arrival. This advocate should also acquaint other staff members with the pertinent information about the new resident.

Once the resident enters the home, the advocate will need to be involved with assisting and befriending the resident. If a meaningful relationship is established, the new resident should feel s/he has a friendly and reliable person who will help in uncertain situations. In assigning an advocate, caution should be exercised so that a proper caring relationship will exist. If a staff member is not sincere in an advocacy role, there could be personal disdain for the new resident. When this occurs, a change in staff advocates should be made immediately. An advocate-resident relationship is highly important to the adjustment of the new resident and must be monitored carefully.

In conjunction with the staff advocate program, a fellow resident **buddy system** should be created. A buddy system operating within the home would allow fellow residents to assist the new resident. Each residential facility has family members who are more adept at socialization than other residents. These individuals should be asked to assist in making their new family member feel at home. Residential staff members should guide this total process in fostering the friendship between the old home members and the new.

Efforts should be made at the earliest possible time to assist the new resident in establishing personal, meaningful relationships with fellow residents. The advocate staff program and buddy system can be combined with activities both within and outside the home to bring the new resident into personal relationships with house members that can be enjoyable and group centered. Including the new resident in residential home activities as soon as possible will help foster a sense of belonging to a family.

Understanding Special Needs

The new resident, a unique individual, brings to this home a special combination of attitudes, desires and values. Staff members must be willing to accommodate the new resident's personal preferences and keep in mind that the resident knows little of this new environment and even less of what the daily expectations are. Staff members need to explain the routine and personal responsibilities that are common to all house members. At the same time, staff must be willing to listen and be understanding of the new resident's responses to these standards. Willingness to listen and communicate with the resident concerning incongruities between his behavior and the existing policy of the home will assist in easing the transition. A dogmatic approach to resident standards early in the placement can turn a promising house member into a rejected and dejected resident.

When residents have deficiencies in expressing personal needs, staff members must be keenly observant of overt behaviors. During these observations and consequent discussions, staff members determine how the resident is adjusting to the home. Accordingly, they must be given opportunities to discuss their observations and note similarities and differences among their recordings. A residential home for persons with unique handicaps needs to be an environment where each resident can achieve a normalized adjustment.

A residence for individuals who have handicaps should regularly review standards within the home. While performing this review, strong consideration must be given to the normalization concept. Examples of residential regulations that commonly surface include:

a   **Smoking habits:** are smoking regulations too rigid? Smoking is hazardous to one's health but not illegal.

b   **Wake-up time on weekends and holidays:** do residents have any rights in considering their own wake-up time?

c   **Going to bed:** do times vary for each resident taking into consideration their personal differences?

d   **Independent travel:** are individual differences taken into consideration?

e   **Alcohol consumption:** do eligible residents have reasonable alcohol consumption rights?

f   **Association with members of the opposite sex:** are there any considerations concerning heterosexual associations within the home and outside the home?

g   **Personal property protection:** are regulations insuring that all residents have personal property rights concerning their possessions?

h   **Time to be by oneself:** are there time allowances when residents can have privacy?

i   **Purchasing rights:** do residents have the right to purchase items based solely on their own personal decision?

Trial Period for New Resident

The assumption is sometimes made that any new resident in a residential home for handicapped individuals will make an adequate adjustment. Even when the adjustment is perceived as inadequate, it is thought that the new resident can somehow be forced into the placement—this type of thinking is unjustified. These individuals are no different than any others where changes in residence are concerned. Sometimes a move is successful and sometimes we must realize that such a placement was a mistake.

Any new resident, therefore, should be on a trial basis in a new home. A new placement needs time to be evaluated. The evaluation concerns both the adequacy of the adjustment in reference to the new resident, as well as the adjustment of family members to the resident. Such a placement fit doesn't have to be a perfect match, but a reasonable harmonious adjustment should prevail. If such an adjustment can't be worked out over a fair period of time, the placement should be terminated.

So that no misunderstanding results from such a residential policy, this trial period for each new resident must be clearly defined to all individuals involved in the move. Such a policy explained and understood by all parties from the beginning will help protect the new resident. If the placement doesn't work out, s/he will still have a home to return to. Keeping open the opportunity for the resident to move out of a situation that is not appropriate eliminates manipulation of the resident and protects the emotional well-being of the individual.

Summary

Individuals with severe handicaps who move from one residence to another experience many different feelings. It is a highly emotional period of time in the life of the individual. A stepwise projection of adjustment activities is illustrated in Figure 5.1. A residential move needs to occur over a gradual period of time and needs to preserve some of the old residence by allowing the individual to transfer belongings from a previous home. It is important to establish personal relationships that help the new resident feel welcome in the new environment and to take into account the special needs of the resident. Relevant information about the new resident should be gathered and evaluated so that personal adjustment problems may be solved. Finally, a trial period should be established to evaluate the appropriateness of the targeted residential setting. A useful checklist follows to facilitate the flow of activities leading toward the successful transitioning from previous living environments.

TRIAL PERIOD

RELEVANT INFORMATION

MEETING SPECIAL NEEDS

MEANINGFUL RELATIONSHIPS

APPRECIATING THE NEW

PRESERVING SOME OF THE OLD

GRADUATED MOVEMENT

Fig. 5.1

New Resident Information

Check List
Have the following actions been taken so as to facilitate the move of the new resident?

A. Has the new resident visited the home?
☐ Yes   ☐ No
Comments:
Suggestions:

B. Have personnel from our home visited the present home of the new resident:
   ☐ Yes   ☐ No
   Comments:
   Suggestions:

C. Has the new resident spent some time with the present residents of the home?
   ☐ Yes   ☐ No
   Comments:
   Suggestions:

D. Has the relevant information concerning the new resident been obtained?
   ☐ Yes   ☐ No
   List information received:
   List information still to be obtained:

E. Did the resident have the opportunity to bring his personal property to the new home?
   ☐ Yes   ☐ No
   Comments:
   Suggestions:

F. Have the new resident's parents or guardian visited him at the new home?
   ☐ Yes   ☐ No
   Comments:
   Suggestions:

G. Has a staff advocate been assigned to the new resident?
   ☐ Yes   ☐ No
   Comments:
   Suggestions:

H. Has documentation been made concerning the new resident's special needs? (e.g., smoking, rides a bicycle, likes to cook)
   ☐ Yes   ☐ No
   Comments:
   Suggestions:

Chapter 6

Voluntary Community Resources

The utilization of volunteer individual assistance has been a major building block in the formation of the democratic society. The early settlers in America, those courageous individuals who, almost out of necessity for survival in their new land, volunteered their time to assist others so that the basic fibers of their new existence could be maintained. The plowing, planting and harvesting of crops, the raising of cabins, homes and barns are only a few examples of how volunteerism, freely giving of one's time without thought of recompense, has played an important part in the early development of this country.

Volunteerism has not weakened in this country from those early days, however, the form it has taken may have changed. Instead of raising a neighbor's barn, American citizens may now assist their neighborhood by volunteering time to work with the senior population of the community by assisting at the community nursing home two nights a week. Or, instead of helping a neighbor harvest his crops, American citizens may now assist their neighborhood by volunteering time to work with community teenagers at the teen center on Friday nights. The strong concept of volunteerism in American life has definitely not weakened—only changed direction.

Volunteerism is a part of American life, however, has it been an effective technique in helping others? Let's answer that question by using an hypothetical situation proposed by Professor Edward C. Lindeman of the New York School of Social Work. In his proposal, all volunteers in this country would go on strike. These individuals would no longer volunteer their service:

> ...all trustees of colleges, universities and private schools; all members of local school boards; all directors of private institutions and agencies; all solicitors for community chests; all lay boards collaborating with public institutions and agencies; all committee members of private institutions and agencies; and that great host of citizens who serve multitudes of educational, welfare, health and recreation organizations in one capacity or another.

One can discern from this hypothetical example that volunteer assistance has been an effective technique for helping others in so many facets of American life. Moreover, and important to this book, voluntary community assistance can be an effective helping technique to individuals involved in the operation of residential facilities for the handicapped.

There are many human resources within communities that can contribute to the positive growth of a residential facility. Volunteers can be included in many facets of the residential home. For example, volunteers could participate in the general operation of the facility as a member of the advisory board or in the direct care programming of the residents as a volunteer direct care worker. The use of auxiliary resource personnel is determined by the specific needs of the home and the ability of the permanent staff of the home to recruit volunteers.

Effective service by these individuals takes careful planning and appropriate judgement by the facility's permanent staff. The staff of the facility must avoid carelessness in the management, selection and monitoring of volunteers. When volunteers are used effectively, the facility benefits tremendously; if used in an inefficient manner, the facility loses.

Few facilities for residents with severe handicaps have the financial resources to adequately meet the many needs of their residents. An organized effort by the facility in the direction of achieving a strong voluntary resource pool can compensate for these financial shortcomings. This chapter will offer suggestions on how to profit from such cost-effective resource personnel.

Coordinator: Volunteer Resource Personnel

The most important consideration in the organizational planning for the implementation of volunteers is to designate a staff member as coordinator. This staff member would be responsible for coordinating all aspects of the volunteer program. When a designated staff member assumes a role as coordinator, a focal point of responsibility exists to insure that coordination doesn't become an elusive matter. Many programs that include volunteer resource assistance fail in their pursuit because no one on the residential staff understands who is responsible for this task. Assign one staff member to coordinate this matter and your residential facility will avoid such a problem.

A primary consideration of the coordinator of volunteers is to be community minded; s/he must be an individual who enjoys being involved in community matters and traveling about the community. This responsibility brings the staff member into contact with diverse individuals and calls for effective people skills. Also, the coordinator will need to be a person who can motivate people to work and ensure that permanent staff develop a positive relationship with the volunteer to their assignments.

The present residential staff may not contain a person who possesses the skills to effectively coordinate a volunteer program. A search should be undertaken to fill this position. A person could be obtained on a voluntary basis or a paid position may need to be established for a personnel resource coordinator.

The personnel coordinator will need to conduct regular meetings with the facility's staff members in conjunction with volunteer staff. These meetings should concentrate on the effectiveness of the overall volunteer program and the specific program benefits that each resident is receiving. The coordinator must operationalize the program objectives and be able to communicate these objectives to facility personnel and volunteer staff. Program objectives must be clearly delineated at these meetings to insure that everyone understands the volunteer resource program and is cooperating so that such a program can be of real assistance to the facility.

The resource personnel coordinator will assume varied responsibilities including the following:

Identify needs of the facility that could benefit from volunteer assistance. The coordinator's keen observation of the actual functioning of the residential facility will uncover certain personnel needs. There exists facility operation areas where budget restraints do not allow for additional staff and where volunteer assistance could be of a real benefit. For example, the programmatic area for the residents, often a real need area, possibly could use a number of volunteers three or four nights a week to assist with the recreational activities in the home.

Identify individuals in the community who would have specific expertise that could meet facility needs. In this area of personnel identification, individuals who have special training are usually sought. For instance, a physician, nurse, minister, dentist and other professionally trained individuals are identified as possible candidates for volunteer assistance to the residential facility.

Delineate specific objectives for each volunteer position. When volunteers enter the facility in an assisting manner, let them clearly understand what their responsibilities are when working for the facility. Write out and carefully explain to each volunteer the duties or responsibilities the facility expects them to perform. Volunteers should not have to wander aimlessly through their volunteer hours wondering what is expected of them.

Solicit assistance from organizations within the community which have needed expertise. Examples of special groups would be the Red Cross, a retired teachers association or the Future Teachers of America organization at the local high school. Many special organizations within the community could have an unique expertise that could possibly benefit the facility from a volunteer standpoint.

Speak to different people in the community who are, or could be, interested in volunteer service. This is the direct approach to securing volunteer community assistance. Staff members from the residential facility can seek volunteer help within the community, speaking at club meetings and other such efforts.

Work with permanent staff to facilitate appropriate blending of the volunteer staff within the facility. Once volunteer help has become a reality within the operations of the facility, insure that permanent staff work in a positive relationship with the volunteer staff. Insure that staff and volunteer roles are understood by all individuals, and that the permanent staff help the volunteers in accomplishing their objectives. Volunteer staff should never be led to feel isolated from permanent staff members or that they are being used but not appreciated by the facility's permanent staff members.

There is no better way to say thanks than to establish a regular volunteer award system for the noncompensated staff members of the facility. An award system can be developed in many ways, from a rather elaborate banquet setting and awards ceremony to a rather simple photograph hanging in the living room of the facility honoring the volunteer of the month. The point being made, however, is not what award system is best, but to establish some regular method of thanking the facility's volunteers.

Work with the volunteer resource personnel in improving their volunteer contribution toward the home. Establish regular meetings with the facility's volunteers. Meetings will help foster open communication with the volunteer staff and, hopefully, create a better informed and trained volunteer staff. In fact, educational workshops, planned for the volunteer staff for the purpose of upgrading volunteer's skills, are highly encouraged as a staff improvement technique.

Facility Needs: Potential Volunteer Assistance

Volunteer resource personnel can be involved in many different aspects of the residential facility's operations. These operational responsibilities will come under the direction of the staff coordinator for volunteer help. A listing of some of the potential areas within a residential facility that could benefit from such volunteer personnel reveals that the vast majority of these responsibilities could be under the direction of the volunteer coordinator. In certain instances, however, like the advisory board member, the coordinator may assist in the selectioin and the soliciting of such individuals, but have little or no supervisory responsibility.

Facility Areas That May Use Volunteer Assistance
Volunteer Resource Coordinator

Special Service	General Operations	Programming
Religious	Advisory Board	Self Help
Psychological	Financial	Leisure Time
Health Care	Medical	Communication

The following sections contain a discussion on specialized areas that can benefit from volunteer resource personnel. The richness of the imagination of the volunteer coordinator and different needs of the residential facility will dictate other potential areas that could receive volunteer assistance.

Residential Advisory Board

Residential Advisory boards are a part of many residential facilities' management plan; although not a necessary component of all residential facilities. Advisory boards, however, are required in facilities that are developed and financed by governmental agencies. These advisory boards serve the facility in an invaluable manner when the board operates as an advocate of the facility and exists for the betterment of the residents.

An example of an advocacy advisory board is when board members keep the normalization needs of the residents in mind when making facility decisions. An advocacy board decision can be a position to purchase a new motor van for the facility rather than having expansive landscaping completed. The reason for this decision: residents can enjoy more beneficial experiences in their community rather than having to stay at home for long periods of time.

Care, therefore, must be exercised in the selection of advisory board members. The selection of board members should be initiated by the residential facility administrator who solicits assistance from additional individuals who have a broader view of the selection process, including the volunteer coordinator. If possible, individuals outside of the facility should be of assistance in the selection process especially if the facility administrator does not have a good knowledge of community members who could serve effectively on an advisory board.

Because of their position and professional expertise, active community leaders should be coveted members of the board. Each new person must be carefully selected based on the complementation with present board members.

Generalizations concerning all residential facility advisory board members will not be made. Each unique residential facility will dictate the importance of board members who can assist the facility. Specialized care facilities, for example, might be more interested in a higher percentage of board members who have a medical background than a family group home setting with minimal health needs.

The following list contains frequently requested members of an advisory board who can, in most instances, make an important contribution to the advisory board.

Type	Expertise
• Parent/Guardian	advocate, of a general nature, for the residents
• Medical	knowledge in the area of the resident's medical needs— physician, nurse, dentist, health personnel
• Special Education/Specialist	knowledge of the field of the handicapped—nature, education, programming, etc.

- Legal   knowledge of the law in relation-
                           ship to the residents and the
                           facility

- Business/Finance   knowledge of the financial and
                           accounting aspects of the facility

- Consumer/Purchasing   knowledge of purchasing a
                           variety of items for the facility
                           at a saving

Proper coordination of a residential advisory board will create a viable functioning adjunct committee to assist the facility. The administrator of the residential facility should be designated as coordinator. As the appointed director of the facility, this coordinator of the residential advisory board should assemble as strong an advisory board as possible. It is not a responsibility that should be taken casually. A strong advisory board can be too valuable an asset to the facility to take a cursory approach to its organization.

In the organization and operation of an advisory board, responsibilities of the coordinator include:

1. Select advisory board members who are willing to express their opinions even though, at the time, such feelings are contrary to the present policies of the program. An advisory board consisting of board members who are always agreeable to the administrative direction of the facility is probably not watching out for the facility.

2. Terminate board members who show little interest and drag on with spotty attendance and mediocre input.

3. Write up an agenda and mail it out to board members at least a week preceding the scheduled meeting. This agenda should set priorities allowing more time for important issues at the beginning of the meeting. If at all possible, keep the number of agenda items reasonably short so as to encourage board member input.

4. Establish a regular board meeting date and time and keep to this commitment. This allows board members to routinely plan in advance for such meetings.

5. Establish a reasonable time limit to each meeting. Board members are usually quite active in their own professions and personal lives and board meetings that linger on will discourage attendance.

6. Provide, if budget allows, some sort of refreshments for each meeting. Such thoughtfulness is a nice way to say thank you for your time.

7. Encourage board members to become involved in varied facets of the residential facility. Invitations to holiday parties, community trips or just a blanket welcome to visit the facility should be offered.

In summary, advisory boards serve a valuable function for residential facilities and should be carefully organized and used. The appropriate use of a residential advisory board is an outstanding example of the contribution that volunteer resource personnel can take to the operation of a residential facility.

Other Resource Personnel

Grandparent Program. Many communities have a volunteer program that includes productive senior citizens in service situations. These senior citizens serve the community in many diverse capacities. By their service they are contributing to the improvement of the quality of life in their community. The organizational name connotes a group of older, sedentary individuals which may serve in a baby-sitting capacity. Nothing could be further from the truth. This organization has been a vital and dynamic service to the programs that they serve.

To obtain the service of a grandparents program, contact your local senior citizens organization. In some localities, the program is associated within another volunteer agency. The grandparents concept may also be referred to by different titles.

When contacting this particular group, be sure and specify the exact nature of your residents' handicapping conditions. There should be no misunderstanding from the beginning that unusual behaviors and conditions can exist in the residents. For example, individuals who have epileptic seizures should be identified and the volunteer taught how to react, so that an attack doesn't become a frightening experience for the volunteer. The coordinator must communicate each residents' unique behavior to the volunteer. This open communication can be programmed so that initial contact with the facility by the volunteers will be accompanied by observation and discussion. One of the purposes of these initial facility contacts is to alleviate unfounded anxieties that a volunteer could have from some previous misunderstanding or lack of knowledge concerning the facility's residents. The communication of meaningful information and the informal association with the residential family can dispel unwarranted volunteer restraint.

Mature individuals with many years of varied experiences are the type of volunteers that are difficult to cultivate. A grandparents organization offers such qualifications at a volunteer's price. The volunteer coordinator should definitely seek out this assistance for the residential facility.

University Programs. Universities and colleges throughout the country have volunteer community service organizations. These student volunteer programs have as their objective to provide service to the local community and to provide college students with the opportunity to gain new challenging experiences in their young lives. Experience has shown that both the community and the students benefit from such a volunteer service. Individuals interested in a volunteer program should contact their local universities or college volunteer student organization.

A more direct approach to soliciting student assistance would be to contact specific university departments. The most important of these university departments would be the Department of Special Education. This specialized department trains university students, who upon graduation, enter professional fields of service in varied areas of education for persons with handicaps. Special education majors have made a professional career commitment and would function in a residential facility in a professional manner. Additional university departments to consider contacting would be the departments of Psychology, Physical Therapy, Occupational Therapy, Sociology, Adaptive Physical Education, Art/Music Therapy, Home Economics and any other specialized areas that could be of benefit to the residents.

Considerations for working with student volunteers include:

1. These are intelligent students; however, the vast majority are between eighteen and twenty-two years of age. Supervisors must be careful in how much and how rapid responsibility is delegated.

2. Direct supervision is necessary so that the university student receives proper guidance.

3. Some university students will need assistance in how to establish relationships with the residents on a mature level, not childlike or authoritylike.

4. Provide adequate in-service training and continuous training for the university students.

5. You will need to be flexible in arranging schedules. University students have a major responsibility to their university coursework; if possible, careful consideration should be given each scheduling request.

6. Policies of the residential facility should be no different for university students than for regular staff members. Policy examples would concern such items as dress code, tardiness, eating and smoking habits.

7. Provide appropriate feedback (evaluation) to the university students. They desire to perform better and frequent feedback will contribute to their continual growth in the area.

University and college student volunteer assistance can be a valuable service to a facility if proper guidance and policies are established.

Other Community Resources. There are, within almost all communities, numerous organizations whose primary purpose is to provide service to their local community. Such service can be people service and/or financial assistance. In providing people service, individuals will volunteer for an opportunity to assist or befriend fellow citizens. Also, many service organizations assist qualified community projects with financial contributions. It is not unusual for service groups to look for worthy projects to fund within their local community.

Information concerning service organizations can be obtained from a community service resource booklet published in many communities. If the source of this publication cannot be located, contact key community individuals to provide guidance in identifying local service organizations. Once service groups are identified, investigate important characteristics of each service organization. A primary characteristic is the service organization's history of providing assistance to specific groups within the community. Evaluate a service organization for their commitment to service projects. A casual commitment is not what you are desiring, but instead a serious commitment of long duration is a greater benefit to the residential facility.

The residential facility will need to reach out to these community organizations. A good approach is to make a presentation to the different service organizations. This presentation should be well organized and present the residential facility in an interesting manner. Often, the best technique is to use a slide/audio format to protray the facility in an interesting visual manner. A presentation is more effective if the majority of slides depict the residents rather than just merely presenting slides of the facility.

If initial contacts with service group volunteers result in positive feedback, select a volunteer coordinator within the service group. This individual will be responsible for organizing the manpower and/or funding requests. Once an individual has been identified, maintain personal contact and establish a working relationship that fosters mutual benefits for both parties.

The following list contains community service organizations that have been of assistance to resident facilities throughout the country:

Knights of Columbis   American Legion
Lions Club   Optomist Club
Shriners   VFW
Hospital Guilds   Church Service Groups
Big Brothers/Big Sisters   Youth Groups

Suggestions for Working with Volunteer Assistance

1. The volunteers should know exactly what service they are to provide.
2. The residential facility's policies should be clearly understood by the volunteers.
3. An in-service training program should be organized for the volunteers.
4. Volunteers who are delinquent in their attendance or service should be advised that future absentism could result in termination of their involvement with the facility.
5. Personal relationships need to be established with the volunteers so that they feel welcome in the facility.
6. The volunteers should be given every opportunity to express their ideas or feelings about the program.
7. A discussion with the permanent staff concerning the service provided by the volunteers should be held on a routine basis by the volunteer coordinator.
8. Frequent feedback should be provided for the volunteers concerning their activity with the residents.
9. Different assignments can be rotated to maintain volunteer interest.
10. The volunteers should feel a part of the home and welcomed to casual and special facility events.
11. Learn as much as you can about the volunteers so that their special skills or talents may be optimally exposed.
12. Evaluate the entire volunteer program on a regular basis.

Organizational Plan for Establishing a Volunteer Program

As previously stated, sound organization is the key to an effective volunteer resource program. The establishment of a volunteer coordinator within the facility is an initial step toward this organization. The following flow of activity is suggested to assemble a sound volunteer system within the residential facility scheme.

Scheme: Organizational Plan

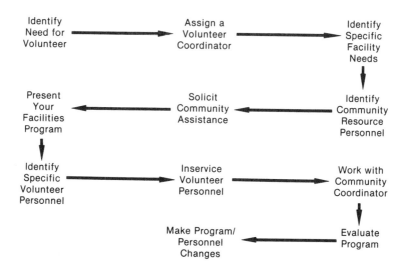

Volunteer Program Forms

There are many forms that can be developed for maintaining volunteer staff programs in a residential facility. Forms can be developed to assist the coordinator in recruiting, training, supervising and evaluating aspects of the volunteer services.

A prime consideration for volunteer program forms is to be able to limit paperwork and not overwhelm the coordinator. At the end of this chapter are four samples of forms that enable the coordinator to distribute and receive pertinent information.

Summary

Residential facilities can benefit tremendously from the service of community resource individuals. If properly coordinated, these community volunteers offer the facility salary-free staff members who can make a valuable contribution to the residential facility. Designating a coordinator is the first objective in planning a volunteer program. The residential facility's specific needs for commnity resource individuals should be identified. Following this identification, resource service individuals can serve on the residential advisory board or provide direct service to the residents of the home. The individuals who volunteer their service to the residential facility may originate from many varied community resources.

Form 1. **Volunteer Manual.** This manual is to be handed out to each volunteer.

Subject Headings
1 List of staff's names and titles
2 List of volunteers
3 Appropriate Dress
4 Job Titles
5 Job Responsibilities
6 Volunteer Check-In Sheet
7 Calling In When You Can't Come In
8 Fire Procedures
9 Emergency Procedures
10 In-service Training Programs

Form 2. Job Description Form for Volunteers
Volunteer's Job Title: _____
Responsible To: _____
Location: _____
Job Responsibility (include general responsibilities as well as specific responsibilities):
_____
_____
_____

Time/Days Required: _____

Required In-service Training _____
_____
_____

In-service Training Provided: _____
_____
_____

Qualifications and Special Skills Needed: _____
_____

Signed: _____

Form 3. Contract for Volunteer Staff

As a volunteer, I _____
will follow the residential facility's policy and procedures as outlined for all
staff members of the facility.

I, _____ , also agree to volunteer
_____ hours a week to the facility; the days I will be here each week are

_____

_____

(other facility considerations can become a part of this contract)

Signed: _____

Volunteer

Date: _____

Form 4. Volunteer Questionnaire Form

1. Do you feel a part of the facility as a volunteer staff member?	yes ☐ no ☐
2. Are your volunteer responsibilities clearly understood?	yes ☐ no ☐
3. Do you feel that you are appreciated by the permanent staff of the facility?	yes ☐ no ☐
4. Are you given enough work to do through out the day?	yes ☐ no ☐
5. Have you been given enough information concerning the residents?	yes ☐ no ☐

(other questions pertaining to your particular facility can be added)

Chapter 7

Instructional Strategies for Conducting Training Programs

The purpose of this chapter is to describe a range of instructional strategies for providing residents with skills to function both within the home and community environments. It is generally recommended that, during training programs, data be collected for the purpose of making decisions relative to program effectiveness. Too much emphasis on data collection can take away from the effectiveness and interaction between the resident and the trainer. However, too little data collection leaves evaluation of progress a questionnable conclusion. The purpose of data collection is to assist the trainer in deciding to continue, modify or terminate the current instructional strategies.

The emphasis in this chapter is not on the data collection procedure itself, but on alternative instructional strategies that should occur when an analysis of data indicates a need to modify an existing program.

Gold (1980) stressed that when an individual fails to learn a task, it is too easy to just say that s/he was incapable of learning the task. Instead, there needs to be a change in focus to provide trainers more power in their teaching strategies to ensure a higher probability of success by the resident. The resident may still eventually not learn the task, but trainers need to exhaust their supply of power before blaming the student for not acquiring a targeted skill.

For organizational purposes, teacher power has been divided into three strategies: Antecedent change, modifying the task, and consequent change. Each of these strategies is detailed in the following sections.

Antecedent Change

Antecedent change refers to the trainer's behavior that occurs prior to the intended response by the resident. thus, antecedents are those events occurring before the resident's behavior that can be arranged to greatly enhance the resident's performance. Two teacher strategies that will be emphasized in this section are prompt hierarchies and time delay.

Prompt Hierarchies

A prompt hierarchy is a system of trainer prompts that is delivered in a contingent manner. That is, the trainer prompts are selected based on each resident's reaction to present cues. A general explanation of typically employed prompts is listed below, followed by a discussion of a least prompting and most prompting cue hierarchy.

Individual Elements of Prompt Hierarchies

Nonspecific Verbal Cue. A general statement of expectation by the trainer to pace the resident through a task.

Example: What's next?
What do you do now?
Please continue.
Next.

Specific Verbal Cue. A statement that details exactly what is to be done by the resident.

Example: Pick up the top section of the napkin.
Put the shoe lace through the loop.
Turn off the cold water.

Pictoral Presentation. Line drawings or photographs representing the intended behavior to be performed by the resident.

Example: Making iced tea (steps #9 & #10 from Bates & Pancsofar, 1979)

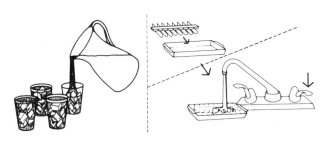

Gesture. A pointing motion to direct the resident to the task relevant cues.

Example: Pointing to the cold water faucet to draw attention to the relevant cue for turning on the cold water.

Model-Demonstration.

a) Miming the correct motions expected by the resident without actually changing the task.

Example: Using a counterclockwise turning motion above the cold water faucet to indicate the desired response of turning on the cold water.

b) Demonstrating the correct steps by actually performing part of the task.

Example: Actually turning on the cold water by moving the faucet in a counterclockwise direction.

Physical Prime. Making slight contact with part of the resident's hand-wrist-arm.

Example: Touching the resident's elbow for one second and applying slight pressure in the direction of the intended activity.

Physical Guidance. Placing trainer's hand on part of resident's hand-wrist-arm and maintaining contact throughout movement of response.

Example: Physically guiding a scooping motion using hand-over-hand assistance during a feeding sequence of steps.

Seven forms of trainer assistance have been delineated in this section. Combinations of assistance strategies can also be used. For example, a nonspecific verbal cue of "What's next?" can be used in combination with a physical prime of a touch on the elbow.

Least Prompting

Least prompting refers to the arrangement of least-to-most amounts of trainer assistance. The purpose for providing trainer assistance in a least prompting manner is for the resident to respond to as many natural cues from the task itself and only provide as little additional artificial information as possible based on the resident's responses. For example, Figure 7.1 contains a progression of three types of trainer assistance (specific verbal cue, gesture combined with a specific verbal cue, and physical guidance combined with a verbal cue). The trainer would follow this sequence when interacting with the resident on a chosen activity. If sufficient progress was not noted, a change in the amount and type of assistance could be included or substituted for in the progression. Another progression might be pictoral cue only, pictoral cue plus modelling, and pictoral cue plus physical guidance (hand-over-hand assistance). Whatever sequence is used, the objective is to present increasingly more intense assistance only after the resident has either incorrectly responded or failed to respond at all to less amounts of information.

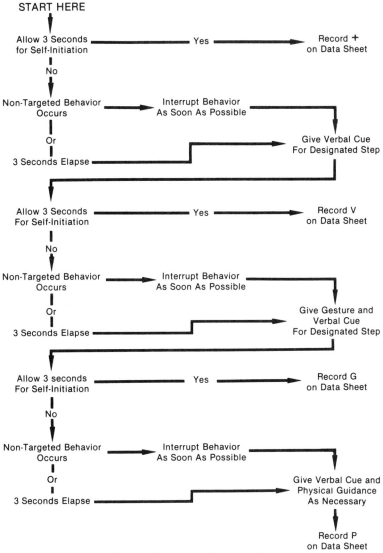

Fig. 7.1 Three Types of Trainer Assistance

Most Prompting

Most prompting contains an arrangement of most to least amounts of trainer assistance. Some steps in a task sequence may be difficult and require initial hand-on-hand assistance with fading as the student initiates more of the movements of the task. A criterion could be set at three correct trials in a row before advancing to less intense prompts. The following sequence presents an arrangement of prompts in a progression from most intense assistance to less intense assistance.

Hand-on-hand assistance

P-1   *Trainer guides resident's hand through the movements of the targeted response with no resident resistance.*

P+1   *Trainer places his/her hand on resident's hand while resident initiates all movements of the targeted response.*

Hand-on-wrist assistance

P-2   *Trainer guides residents wrist through the movements ot the targeted response.*

P+2   *Trainer places his/her hands on resident's wrist while resident initiates all movements of the targeted response.*

Hand-on-forearm assistance

P-3   *Trainer guides resident's forearm through movements of the targeted response.*

P+3   *Trainer places his/her hand on resident's foremarm while resident initiates all movements of the targeted respoonse.*

Hand-on-elbow assistance

P-4   *Trainer guides resident's elbow through the movement of the targeted response.*

P+4   *Trainer places his/her hand on resident's elbow while resident initiates all movements kof the targeted response.*

Hand-on-upper arm assistance

P-5   *Trainer guides resident's upper arm through the movements of targeted response.*

P+5 *Trainer places his/her hand on resident's upper arm while resident initiates all movements of the targeted response.*

A progression of trainer assistance from P-1 through P+5 does not entail moving in a rigid sequence order of P-1, P+1, P-2, P+2, ...P+5. Instead, representative options from the ten strategies could be sequenced such as P-1, P+1, P+3, and P+5. It is extremely difficult to delineate the subtleties of working with unique individuals and knowing when to release pressure or how to describe degrees of pressure that are applied to help assist residents through movements of the targeted response.

Time Delay

Time delay is an antecedent strategy whereby natural and artificial cues are presented simultaneously and then the latency of presentation of the artificial cue gradually increases over time. An example would be the following. The requested task might be the resident's request (via signing) for a glass of orange juice when presented with the natural cue of a full glass of orange juice. Initially, the trainer would present the full glass and simultaneously give the artificial cue of a model of the correct sign. If the resident could sufficiently imitate the sign, s/he could then receive the orange juice. A few trials later, the trainer would present the full glass of orange juice (natural cue) to the resident and wait one-half to one second before presenting the modeled sign (artificial cue). After a pre-determined number of successful signs, the trainer would rpesent the glass of juice and wait two full seconds before revealing the modeled cue. Present research suggests that after four to five seconds of latency the resident will begin anticipating that a response is required by the natural cue before the previously required artificial cue is given. For a more detailed discussion on the use of time delay the reader is referred to Billingsley and Romer (1983), Halle, Marshall, and Spradlin (1979), Snell (1982), and Snell and Gast (1981).

Modifying the Task Presentation

Modifying the task presentation refers to trainers providing assistance strategies that focus on alternative ways of presenting the task to the resident in order to facilitate skill acquisition. The two sample strategies that are described in this section are Chaining and Color Cue Redundancy.

Chaining

Chaining refers to the presentation of a sequenced order of small steps that are linked together to form a more complex network of steps to acquire a targeted skill. Bates and Pancsofar (1981b) describe three chaining techniques: Teach all, forward, backward.

Residents with severely handicapping conditions learn more efficiently if the tasks to be learned are presented in smaller units of behavior. With task analysis, component steps of specific tasks are delineated. One technique for conducting instruction with task analysis is to provide specific training on all steps in the task. In this "teach all" technique, the trainer instructs the resident on all steps of a task that are not independently performed. For many individuals, this technique will be effective. However, if a resident does not learn quickly with this method, techniques involving instruction of only one step at a time should be considered.

In one of these methods, the trainer teaches the resident to initially perform the behavior required in the first step of the task analysis. No other teaching would take place until the resident acquired the ability to perform this first step. Once the resident performed step one, the trainer would now require the resident to complete step one and begin work on step two. As the resident learned how to follow each new step, the behavior chain would be lengthened until the resident performed all steps in this task analysis. An advantage of this technique is that the resident is required to learn only one step at a time. For very slow learning residents, this practice may be necessary to insure acquisition.

Another type of chaining technique also involves teaching the resident to complete one step at a time, proceeding from the first to the last. However, with this technique, the resident is physically assisted to complete the entire task after receiving instruction on the first step. After completing the first step, the trainer provides assistance on step two and continues with physical assistance for the remaining steps. This procedure continues through the remaining steps.

The previously presented chaining strategies were variations of forward chaining. Two additional chaining techniques that may prove useful for facilitating skill acquisition are backward chaining methods.

In the first method, the trainer assists the resident through the steps of the task analysis just prior to where the resident can complete the task on his/her own. Instruction is conducted on this one step. After the training session on this sequence is finished, the resident is allowed to finish the task. As the resident acquires the skills required in this chain of the task, the trainer would physically assist the resident through less and less of the task.

The second type of backward chaining is identical to the above method with the exception that the trainer prepares the first part of the task on his/her own rather than physically assisting the resident. Both of these methods are similar in that they only require the resident to learn one step at a time leading toward acquisition of the entire skill. (pp. 14-17)

Adding and Fading of a Color Cue

Another instructional program that was described by Bates and Pancsofar (1981a) contained an example of modifying the task by adding a redundant color cue to the task. The activity was folding and stacking linen towels in a work setting at a county hospital. The task analysis included the following steps:

1. Pick up one unfolded hand towel from pile of hand towels on folding table.
2. Shake/straighten towel if necessary.
3. Place towel on table in rectangular form—long edge nearest to worker.
4. Using thumb and fingers of each hand, pick up either two right edges or two left edges of towel.
5. Fold towel by bringing top edge across to touch opposite top edge and bottom edge across to touch opposite bottom edge.
6. Match corners so there is no overlap and corners are even.
7. Using thumb and fingers of each hand, grasp either the top two edges or the bottom edges of towel.
8. Fold towel by bringing right edge across to touch opposite right edge and left edge across to touch opposite left edge.
9. Match corners so there is no overlap and corners are even.
10. Using thumb and fingers of each hand, grasp each edge of the single fold side of towel.
11. Pick up towel.
12. Place towel on stack of folded towels so that the single fold edge of towel is placed on the top towel's nonfold side.
13. Repeat steps 1-12 for remaining towels in unfolded stack.

A baseline assessment of the 13 steps of the task analysis was conducted by the trainer. During baseline, the worker independently completed nine of the thirteen steps. Initial training consisted of least prompting assistance with a direction-demonstration-physical guidance sequence. After one week of this assistance, three additional steps of the task analysis were completed independently. Step 12, the process of folding towels so that the single fold edge of the recently folded towel is placed on top towel's nonfold side, was still not being performed independently. The purpose for stacking folded towels in the manner detailed in Step 12 was for efficient storage in the hospital's towel closets (i.e., more towels could be placed on top of each other if the towels were alternately stacked).

Since least prompting did not provide a powerful enough assistance, the trainer decided to include a second training strategy, that consisted of adding and fading of a color cue. The color cue that was provided for this activity was a black highlighted line placed on the seam of the nonfold edge of the training towel. This color-coded seam would provide the worker with a visual cue for where to place the single fold edge of the most recently folded towel. After the worker correctly placed the towel on the highlighted seam the trainer would remove the training towel, replace it on top of the stack, and have the seam facing the opposite direction. Thus, the worker alternated towels on the stack while responding to the redundant color cue. As the worker began to consistently place the folded towel on the correct part of the training towel, the highlighted cue was faded. The fading sequence is shown in Figure 7.2. After three days of using the color cue fading process combined with a least prompting strategy, the worker was correctly stacking the towels to accomplish the specific program objective.

Fading Nonessential Cue

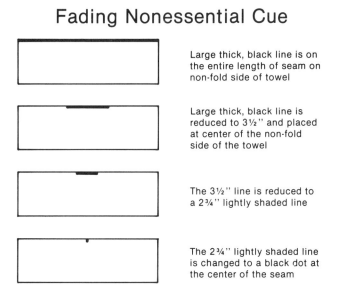

Large thick, black line is on the entire length of seam on non-fold side of towel

Large thick, black line is reduced to 3½" and placed at center of the non-fold side of the towel

The 3½" line is reduced to a 2¾" lightly shaded line

The 2¾" lightly shaded line is changed to a black dot at the center of the seam

Fig. 7.2

Consequent Changes

Consequent events that will be described in this section are those resident and trainer behaviors that reinforce the resident's completion of a targeted response or chain of responses. That is, a reinforcer is any event which, when presented, increases the probability of a response it follows. Events, in and of themselves, cannot be considered reinforcers unless they increase the future probability of the behavior that they follow. Figure 7.3 presents a hierarchy of reinforcement options available to the trainer. The arrangement of reinforcers progresses from a basic level (primary reinforcers) to a more advanced level (self-reinforcers).

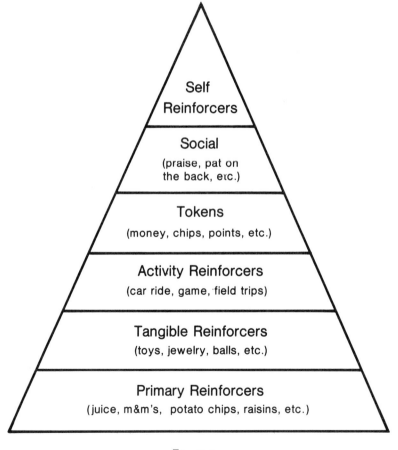

Fig. 7.3

Bates and Pancsofar (1981b) summarized each of the reinforcement options contained in Figure 7.3.

A primary reinforcer is a substance that requires no learning by the resident in order for it to have reinforcing properties. Juice, candy, raisins, and soda may be such items. A tangible reinforcer is an object that is of preference by the resident that s/he can manipulate for a short period of time. Activity reinforcers are preference behaviors such as games, listening to music, going for a walk, or going on a field trip. A token is a "tangible object which serves as a generalized conditioned reinforcer. It can be exchanged for a backup reinforcer from which it derives its value." (Kazdin, 1980, p. 368) A social reinforcer is an interpersonal encounter with other individuals which results in an increase in the behavior it follows. Verbal praise, pats on the back, and attention are common social reinforcers. Self-reinforcers are delivered by the resident and may include verbal self-praise, or self-administering of a token, activity, tangible, or primary reinforcer.

During skill acquisition, reinforcers should be administered on a continuous basis. Reinforcers should be delivered immediately and with enthusiasm. At all times higher order reinforcers (e.g., social praise) should be paired with more basic reinforcers (e.g., tokens). As residents acquire new skills, the schedule of delivery should become more intermittent and natural reinforcers should be established.

In order to maintain an updated list of potential reinforcers for each resident, it is suggested that a resident reinforcement survey be obtained. A sample survey follows.

Resident Reinforcement Survey

The objective of this survey is to ensure that the resident is receiving feedback at the most appropriate level of reinforcement at this time. Progress toward this objective can be assessed by the trainer by specifying type(s) of reinforcers and how often each reinforcer is being utilized in the resident's training programs.

Please list those specific reinforcers being currently used for this resident under the appropriate categories. Beside each listed reinforcer specify whether the reinforcer is being used continuously (c) or intermittently (i). For example, if a sip of juice is given after each correct response on a color matching task, this would be listed as juice (c) under Primary Reinforcers. Or if the opportunity to listen to several minutes of music is given after washing the evening dishes, this would be listed as listening to music (i) under Activity Reinforcers. Please keep in mind that a reinforcer is anything that one is willing to exert some effort to obtain. Most importantly, a reinforcer is solely defined by its effect on the behavior that it follows; it increases the probability that the behavior will occur again.

Primary Reinforcers: Those things which are not learned and maintain/perpetuate life, e.g., food, water, warmth.

Concrete Reinforcers: Those things which are learned and can be manipulated, e.g., toys, clay, trinkets, books.

Activity Reinforcers: Those things which are learned and are preferred activities, e.g., listening to music, water play, singing, going shopping.

Token Reinforcers: Those things which are learned and can be exchanged, e.g. money, chips, points for activity reinforcers.

Social Reinforcers: Those things which are learned and are those forms of positive attention that one person provides another person, indicating approval, e.g., spoken words such as "Great, I'm so proud of you"; facial expressions such as smiling, nodding; or bodily expressions such as patting on the back, hugging, shaking hands.

Intrinsic Reinforcers: Those things which are learned and involve feelings of satisfaction in accomplishing a task, e.g., working on a task due to one's interest or enjoyment in performing the task.

Summary

Included in this chapter were three suggested approaches to increase the probability that residents will learn targeted behaviors. Examples of antecedent and consequent changes as well as modifying the components of the task itself were provided. Used in isolation or in combination, these strategies contain ways to increase trainer power when teaching residents who find it difficult to learn through more informal instruction. A combination of the three strategies should provide the trainer with a multitude of prompting sequences. The trainer must keep in mind that the ultimate goal is to shift the stimulus control from artificially imposed cues to the natural task relevant cues that are presented to the resident in the absence of the trainer's assistance. Thus, we can realize Gold's (1980) caution not to blame the learner for failure but to question the power of our training strategies.

Chapter *8*

Domestic Living Skills

Domestic living skills refer to the array of behaviors necessary to function as independently as possible within a home setting. Complete independence in all home living skills is not an ultimate goal for severely handicapped residents. Independence is better explained as a function of environmental opportunities and demands, modification in those demands, individual skills, and the daily application of those skills (Vogelsberg, Williams, and Bellamy, 1982). The rationale for selecting new skills for severely handicapped residents must be predicated on a thorough search for essential skills that are necessary to function successfully in existing and planned for alternative living environments. More options will become available only when residents are afforded a training curriculum that contains a sequence of designated activities that will assist in meeting current and subsequent demands. The goals of this chapter are to a) develop an orientation of current and subsequent environment strategies and b) establish a data bank of state of the art resources in the domain of domestic living.

Current and Subsequent Domestic Living Inventories

Brown, Branston-McClean, Baumgart, Vincent, Falvey, and Schroeder (1979) provide an outline for determining the range of behaviors that need to be acquired by severely handicapped individuals to successfully function in both a current and future residential settings. To smooth foreseeable transitions from present to subsequent living environments, behavior should be taught to residents that not only enhance current functioning levels but also increase the probability that movement to less restrictive community settings will occur as well. Brown et al. (1979) recommended that a home setting be divided into several subenvironments. With each subenvironment, activities will be delineated that are necessary to effectively function as independently as possible. Specific skills are then listed for each designated activity. Bates and Pancsofar (1981b) illustrate one procedure for following the outline proposed by Brown et al. (1979). In figure 8.1, a range of living option is placed on a continuum of existing residential environments for the handicapped within a specific geographic area. Presently, a person may be residing in a cottage type setting with nine peers on an institution's grounds (option #4 on continuum). However, future placement within the community is foreseeable in a small group home of six to eight residents (option #6 in Figure 8.1). According to Brown et al. (1979), after determining a realistic future-living option, plans must be made to currently teach those skills that are to be expected to occur in that future setting. Accordingly, future option #6 is now divided into major subenvironments of the kitchen, living room, dining room, bedroom, bathroom, and utility room. Figure 8.2 contains the major subenvironments within a possible group home and additionally contains a list of frequently observed activities that residents are expected to participate in as independently as possible. Developing the analysis futher, Figure 8.3 includes a list of behaviors that are specifically required to perform activities that were delineated within the kitchen subenvironment. If this analysis were continued for each subenvironment of an option #6 group home, a list of targeted behaviors would be developed for the resident in option #4 that would smooth the transition for a more appropriate future residential placement as a result of the acquisition of preselected, functional domestic living.

Domestic Living Skills

1	2	3	4	5	6	7	8	9	10

Institution	Group Home	Apartment

Continuum of Home Living Environments

1. Large Isolated Institution: dormitory style living
2. Community Residential Facilities: 2 to 3 persons per room but 80 to 100 total residents at facility
3. Institution: cottage living with less than 20 residents per cottage
4. Institutions: cottage living with less than 10 residents per cottage
5. Large Community Group Home: 8 to 16 residents per group home
6. Small Group Home: 6 to 8 residents per group home
7. Foster Home: less than 6 residents
8. Transitional Apartment Group Homes: less than 6 residents
9. Supervised Apartment Living
10. Independent Apartment Living

Figure 8.1 Continuum of Home Living Environments

Group Home
6-8 residents

Kitchen	Living room	Dining room	Bedroom	Bathroom	Utility room
• preparing meals and snacks • dish-washing • cleaning up • putting food away	• relaxing • music • recreation • looking at books • upkeep of room • dancing • excercis-ing	• meal skills • snack • commu-nication • table games • adult edu-cation classes	• making bed • getting ready for bed • dressing skills • putting clothes away	• hygiene • toileting • cleaning room	• washing & drying clothes • folding clothes • ironing clothes

Fig. 8.2

Kitchen

Preparing meals and snacks	Dishwashing	Cleaning up	Putting food away
training involves:	*training involves:*	*training involves:*	*training involves:*
• ability to prepare meal from cookbook for:	• washing dishes at sink	• use of broom and dust pan	• knowing where food is stored
a) Breakfast	• use of dishwasher	• use of sponge mop	• returning food to proper storage
b) Lunch	• drying dishes	• use of mop	
c) Dinner	• putting clean dishes away		
d) Snack			
• preparing drinks			
a) Tea			
b) Coffee			
c) Cocoa			
d) Juice			
• use of kitchen utensils			
• use of stove			

Fig. 8.3

A second example of an environmental analysis contains a more detailed description of required skills within one domestic skills area, namely, household cleaning. A trainer observed the cleaning activities that typically occur within a small group home. Again, she divided the home into five major subenvironments: kitchen, bathroom, laundry room, family room, and bedroom. Five cleaning tasks were then recorded for each subenvironment. (More tasks could certainly be observed but five for each subenvironment will adequately illustrate this procedure). Subsequently, the trainer delineated five specific skills that needed to be acquired by the resident to successfully complete the cleaning activity. Thus, the environmental analysis follows a detailed compilation of skills that can be observed in a residential environment that may currently exist for a severely handicapped person or that is the next most logical relevant living environment.

Environmental Analysis for Household Cleaning Tasks

A. Kitchen
  1. Wash dishes
     a. Is able to discriminiate between clean and dirty dishes
     b. Is able to adjust water temperature
     c. Is able to tell when soap is off of dishes
     d. Is able to tell when dishes are dry
     e. Is able to discriminate between knives and forks for drawer replacement
  2. Wash floor
     a. Is able to discriminate between clean and dirty floor
     b. Is able to move furniture to another room
     c. Is able to adjust water temperature
     d. Is able to use appropriate amount of detergent
     e. Is able to distinguish when floor is dry
  3. Clean oven
     a. Is able to locate the oven
     b. Is able to take the cap off the oven cleaner
     c. Is able to read the instructions on the can of oven cleaner
     d. Is able to put the rubber gloves on the appropriate hands
     e. Is able to tell time to wait until removal of cleaner
  4. Clean out refrigerator
     a. Is able to open Tupperware containers
     b. Is able to discriminate between usable and spoiled food
     c. Is able to discriminate between fruits and vegetables
     d. Is able to discard spoiled food in proper receptacle
     e. Is able to properly close all containers
  5. Clean out cupboards
     a. Is able to tell when cupboards need to be cleaned out
     b. Is able to remove all items from the cupboard
     c. Is able to discriminate between those items that should be kept and those items that should be discarded
     d. Is able to tell when shelf paper needs replacement
     e. Is able to smooth out all air pockets in freshly laid shelf paper

B. Bathroom
  1. Scrub bathtub
     a. Is able to discriminate bath mat from the rest of the tub
     b. Is able to read directions on tile cleaner
     c. Is able to adjust water temperature
     d. Is able to discriminate between a clean and a dirty bathtub
     e. Is able to replace bath mat into the same location where it was found
  2. Scrub sink
     a. Is able to read directions on tile cleaner
     b. Is able to remove cap off of tile cleaner
     c. Is able to adjust water temperature
     d. Is able to discriminate between a clean and a dirty sink

    e.   Is able to replace toothbrushes in the proper holders
  3. Scrub toilet bowl
    a.   Is able to discriminate between a clean and a dirty toilet bowl
    b.   Is able to discriminate between the toilet lid and seat
    c.   Is able to read directions on toilet cleaner
    d.   Is able to pour in appropriate amount of toilet cleaner
    e.   Is able to flush toilet when finished scrubbing
  4. Clean out medicine cabinet
    a.   Is able to move small objects
    b.   Is able to wipe off small objects
    c.   Is able to tell when medicine should be discarded
    d.   Is able to replace items onto the appropriate shelves
    e.   Is able to read the labels on bottles for sorting purposes
  5. Wash floor
    a.   Is able to discriminate between a clean and a dirty floor
    b.   Is able to adjust water temperature
    c.   Is able to read directions on the detergent bottle
    d.   Is able to use appropriate amount of detergent
    e.   Is able to distinguish when the floor is dry

C. Laundry Room
  1. Sort clothes
    a.   Is able to discriminate between white, light, and dark colored clothes
    b.   Is able to discriminate between machine washable and hand washable clothes
    c.   Is able to discriminate between those clothes to be washed in hot, warm and cold water
    d.   Is able to discriminate between clean and dirty clothes
    e.   Is able to empty all pockets
  2. Load and start washer
    a.   Is able to load clothes in appropriate place in washer
    b.   Is able to read instruction on laundry detergent
    c.   Is able to add appropriate amount of detergent
    d.   Is able to select appropriate cycle
    e.   Is able to turn washer on
  3. Load and start dryer
    a.   Is able to load clothes in appropriate place in dryer
    b.   Is able to tear off a sheet of Bounce and place in dryer
    c.   Is able to select appropriate time and heat setting
    d.   Is able to turn dryer on
    e.   Is able to discriminate between wet and dry clothes
  4. Fold clothes
    a.   Is able to straighten a collar on a shirt
    b.   Is able to hang a dress on a hanger
    c.   Is able to hang a pair of slacks on a hanger
    d.   Is able to distinguish between a sleeve and a collar
    e.   Is able to fold a towel in half

5. Iron clothes
   a. Is able to turn iron on
   b. Is able to select appropriate heat setting
   c. Is able to place a shirt on the ironing board
   d. Is able to spray the appropriate amount of starch
   e. Is able to put a crease in a pair of slacks

D. Family Room
   1. Dust
      a. Is able to discriminate between a clean and a dusty table
      b. Is able to move small objects
      c. Is able to wipe off small objects
      d. Is able to read directions on a can of furniture polish
      e. Is able to replace small objects to their appropriate positions
   2. Vacuum furniture
      a. Is able to distinguish between a couch and couch cushions
      b. Is able to turn vacuum cleaner on
      c. Is able to discriminate between a clean and a dirty couch
      d. Is able to determine which vacuum cleaner attachment to use
      e. Is able to replace cushions to their appropriate positions
   3. Wash windows
      a. Is able to discriminate between clean and dirty windows
      b. Is able to spray appropriate amount of window cleaner on window
      c. Is able to move shades, curtains, and any other objects away from window to be cleaned
      d. Is able to wipe off cleaner without streaking
      e. Is able to replace shades, curtains, and other objects to their proper positions
   4. Wash walls
      a. Is able to discriminate between clean and dirty walls
      b. Is able to move heavy objects away from walls
      c. Is able to adjust water temperature
      d. Is able to add appropriate amount of detergent
      e. Is able to replace any pictures to appropriate positions
   5. Vacuum carpeting
      a. Is able to move heavy furniture
      b. Is able to turn vacuum cleaner on
      c. Is able to determine which vacuum cleaner setting to use
      d. Is able to discriminate between a clean and a dirty carpet
      e. Is able to replace furniture to appropriate positions

E. Bedroom
   1. Make up bed
      a. Is able to determine when to put on clean sheets
      b. Is able to discriminate between fitted and top sheet
      c. Is able to discriminate between top sheet and spread
      d. Knows which way to hold pillow when putting on pillow case

   e. Is able to spread out all ruffles from the sheets, blankets, and spread
2. Dust
   a. Is able to remove small objects from top of dresser
   b. Is able to discriminate between a clean and dusty dresser
   c. Is able to wipe off small objects
   e. Is able to wipe off polish to obtain a shine
3. Sweep carpets
   a. Is able to turn on vacuum
   b. Is able to discriminate between carpets and floor
   c. Is able to choose appropriate vacuum attachment
   d. Is able to choose appropriate vacuum setting
   e. Is able to discriminate between clean and dirty carpets
4. Mop the floor
   a. Is able to discriminate between clean and dirty floor
   b. Is able to remove any carpet
   c. Is able to move heavy furniture
   d. Is able to identify and locate a dust mop
   e. Is able to replace heavy furniture to its proper location
5. Wax the floor
   a. Is able to read directions on floor wax bottle
   b. Is able to apply appropriate amount of wax
   c. Is able to tell time to allow wax to dry
   d. Is able to identify and locate a floor buffer
   e. Is able to turn on buffer

A third example for determining targeted domestic living skills for residents to smoothly exit from more restrictive to less restrictive settings is sampling the priority of Group Home trainers in selected skill areas.

Safety Needs for Group Home Residents

In addition to household cleaning activities, safety skills are an extremely critical targeted area of concentration. Individuals with severely handicapping conditions need assistance to develop adequate safety behaviors. Emphasizing this point, Baker (1979) describes a severely handicapped person as "one whose ability to provide for his or her own basic life sustaining and safety needs is so limited relative to their proficiency expected on the basis of chronological age that it could pose a serious threat to his or her survival." (p. 60) To help reduce this "threat to survival," an emphasis on safety behaviors needs to surface in the residential educational programming.

One means to address this deficit area is to determine the

behaviors that are necessary to survive safely in several community environments. One prominent environment is the resident's present home setting. The primary care provider can describe to the trainer those behaviors which inhibit independent participation in activities at home. Additionally, the trainer should also be concentrating his or her objectives for future potentially available living environments as well. A potential environment might be a smaller group home for individuals with severely handicapping conditions. Group home staff could complete a survey of safety behaviors and establish its degree of importance in that home.

In the Safety Needs survey, a group home is divided into several environments including the kitchen, bathroom, bedroom, living room and outside areas as well as categories for mobility and general safety behaviors. Within each division, safety behaviors are delineated and a rating is used to establish the importance of the acquisition of each safety behavior by the residents. After receiving the information form the safety survey, the residential trainer can select the essential behaviors and develop assessment situations to evaluate a resident's performance in these areas. Subsequently, behavioral objectives could be developed for skills that are not presently in the resident's repertoire. Using this approach, the trainer is better preparing his or her residents to successfully meet the demands of a future environment and help insure acceptance as an appropriately functioning resident.

Safety Needs Survey

Included below are several safety behaviors that may or may not be of importance for your residents. Please read each statement and place a number in the blank beside each statement that corresponds to:

    1 = This behavior is not important for the residents to possess

    2 = This is an IMPORTANT behavior for residents to possess in this group home

    3 = This is an ESSENTIAL behavior for residents to possess in this group home

  NA = This behavior does not apply to the residents of this group home

Kitchen Area

_____ carrying hot items
_____ checking expiration date on foods
_____ cleaning appliances safely
_____ covering leftovers properly
_____ cutting foods on appropriate surface
_____ freezing food properly

_____ handling knives and other sharp objects
_____ identifying foods
_____ keeping meltable objects away from heat (styrofoam, bread wrappers, etc.)
_____ operating the stove
    _____ cleaning the oven
    _____ keeping hands away from hot burners
    _____ lighting the pilot light
    _____ placing flammable objects away from heat
    _____ positioning pot handles correctly
    _____ turning off burners when finished
    _____ using appropriate settings for stove and oven
_____ plugging in appliance
_____ pouring hot liquids
_____ recognizing spoiled foods
_____ transporting hot grease
_____ using electrical appliances
    _____ keeping fingers away from beaters on a mixer
    _____ operating popcorn popper
    _____ removing toast that is stuck in toaster
_____ using garbage disposal
_____ using mitts to remove hot items
_____ others

_____
_____
_____

Bathroom Area

_____ adjusting water temperatures
_____ entering and exiting bathtub
_____ no standing in the tub
_____ not leaving soap on shower floor
_____ operating appliances away from water
_____ properly storing medicines
_____ properly using electrical appliance
_____ reading medicine labels
_____ shaving without cutting self
_____ using bathmat in bathtub
_____ using toilet bowl cleaner and other caustic materials
_____ wiping up spilled water
_____ others

_____
_____
_____

Bedroom Area

_____ getting in and out of bed from wheelchair
_____ no cooking in bedroom
_____ no smoking in bed
_____ portable fan operation
_____ others

_____
_____
_____

Living Room Area

_____ adequately building fire in fireplace
        _____ placing protective screen in front of fire
_____ answering the door to strangers
_____ controlling thermostat
_____ keeping area clutter-free
_____ not putting fingers in the fan
_____ returning recreation/leisure materials to proper storage
_____ using scissors
_____ others

_____
_____
_____

Outside Area

_____ changing flat tires
_____ opening garage door before starting car
_____ operating the lawn mower
        _____ cleaning lawn of obstacles
        _____ keeping hands clear of blades
        _____ wearing proper footwear
_____ operating outside grill
_____ recognizing rules of privacy of neighbors
_____ removing snow and ice
_____ riding in auto/van with use of seat belts
_____ shutting door of auto/van
_____ staying in own yard
_____ summoning help from neighbors, if needed
_____ using gardening tools safely
_____ using a stepladder
_____ using insect spray
_____ using safety goggles when working with power tools
_____ other

_____

_____

General Safety Behaviors

_____ administering first aid
    _____ bandaging cuts
    _____ choking procedures
    _____ washing cuts
_____ changing light bulb
    _____ turning off switch
    _____ using dry hands
_____ cleaning up broken glass or other breakage
_____ consuming alcoholic beverages
_____ discriminating between poisons and safe products
_____ evacuating house in event of fire alarm
_____ locking doors at night
_____ making emergency telephone calls to operator, fire station, and/or
        police station
_____ not interfering with someone having a seizure
_____ operating a fire extinguisher
_____ operating the furnace
    _____ activating emergency turn-off
    _____ lighting the pilot light
_____ placing breakable items safely
_____ placing electrical cords to avoid trips/fires
_____ plugging in electrical appliances
    _____ checking cords for wear
    _____ checking for overload
    _____ unplugging appliances after use
    _____ using dry hands
_____ replacing fuses
_____ securing loose rugs/carpets
_____ smoking cigarettes/cigars/pipes
_____ storing papers and rags properly
_____ tornado procedures
_____ using appliances correctly
    _____ iron
    _____ vacuum
    _____ washer/dryer
_____ using candles in the home
_____ using caution on recently waxed floors
_____ using matches or a lighter
_____ utilizing birth control procedures
_____ other

_____

Mobility Area

_____ carrying identification
_____ not leaving objects on stairway
_____ not running in halls
_____ properly crossing streets
_____ recognizing danger signs in community
_____ refusing rides with strangers
_____ using bannisters on stairway
_____ walking at night only in groups of two or more persons
_____ walking on icy outside surfaces
_____ walking on wet surfaces
_____ wearing appropriate clothing to suit the weather
_____ wiping feet upon entering home
_____ other

Domestic Domain

School programs can assist in the acquisition of functional skills within the domestic living domain. A model effort in this direction has been initiated by Bates and Barcus (1982) in Columbia, South Carolina. Twenty-eight objectives were determined by staff to be critical to successful functioning in the domestic domain area. Performance indicators were then listed beneath each objective to evaluate the number of activities that have been completed in order to successfully demonstrate competence for the overall objective.

The domestic domain of the Richland County Curriculum is contained in the following section.

Domestic Domain
Objectives/Performance Indicators

1. Students Should Be Able To Demonstrate Appropriate Bathing Skills.
Performance Indicators
Levels:
I   A.   Turns on water.
      B.   Washes hands.

<pre>
          C.   Dries hands.
          D.   Washes face.
          E.   Dries face.
II   F.   Washes underarms.
          G.   Puts on deodorant
          H.   Takes sponge bath.
III   I.   Adjusts water temperature.
          J.   Takes shower.
          K.   Dries after shower.
          L.   Applies cologne or perfume appropriately.
</pre>

2. Students Should Be Able To Perform Hair Care Skills

Performance Indicators
Level:

<pre>
I   A.   Brushes hair.
          B.   Combs hair.
II   C.   Shampoos hair.
          D.   Uses cream rinse/conditioner.
          E.   Towel dries hair.
          F.   Uses hair dryer.
III   G.   Uses hair rollers (if appropriate).
          H.   Styles hair.
          I.   Washes comb and brush.
</pre>

3. Students Should Be Able To Perform Proper Dental Hygiene.

Performance Indicators

<pre>
I   A.   Brushes teeth.
          B.   Rinses mouth.
II   C.   Flosses teeth.
          D.   Recognizes the need to go to the dentist.
</pre>

4. Students Should Be Able To Perform Proper Nasal Hygiene.

Performance Indicators

<pre>
          A.   Wipes nose with tissue.
          B.   Disposes of used tissue.
          C.   Blows nose with tissue.
          D.   Recognizes when and where nasal care is necessary.
</pre>

5. Students Should Be Able To Perform Proper Shaving Skills.

Performance Indicators

<pre>
          A.   Shaves with electric razor.
          B.   Shaves with safety razor.
          C.   Knows how to use shaving cream or pre-electric shave and
               after-shave.
</pre>

6. Students Should Be Able To Perform Proper Skin Care

Performance Indicators

<pre>
          A.   Uses hand/body lotion.
</pre>

B. Uses acne medication.
C. Recognizes need to wash face.

7. Students Should Be Able To Perform Proper Nail Care
Performance Indicators
Levels:
I   A. Clips nails with clippers.
     B. Files nails.
II   C. Cleans nails with cleaner.
     D. Scrubs nails with brush.
III E. Pushes back cuticles.
     F. Applies nail polish.

8. Students Should Be Able To Perform Proper Feminine Hygiene
Performance Indicators
A. Uses sanitary napkins or tampons.
B. Recognizes when to change napkins or tampons.
C. Disposes of napkins or tampons.
D. Washes and/or uses feminine deodorants.

9. Students Should Be Able To Take Off Clothing Without Fasteners
Performance Indicators
A. Takes off socks.
B. Takes off underwear.
C. Takes off pullover shirts.
D. Takes off clothing with elastic (ex.: pants).
E. Takes off slip-on shoes.

10. Students Should Be Able To Take Off Clothing With Fasteners
Performance Indicators
A. Takes off clothing with zippers.
B. Takes off clothing with buttons.
C. Takes off clothing with snaps.
D. Takes off clothing with hooks and eyes.
E. Takes off clothing with buckles.
F. Takes off shoes with buckles and/or laces.

11. Students Should Be Able To Put On Clothing With No Fasteners
Performance Indicators
A. Put on socks.
B. Put on underwear.
C. Put on pullover shirts.
D. Put on clothing with elastic (ex.: pants).
E. Put on slip-on shoes.

12. Students Should Be Able To Put on Clothing with Fasteners.
Performance Indicators
A. Puts on clothing with zippers.

    B.   Puts on clothing with buttons.
    C.   Puts on clothing with snaps.
    D.   Puts on clothing with hooks and eyes.
    E.   Puts on clothing with buckles.
    F.   Puts on shoes with buckles and/or laces.
    G.   Puts on jackets and coats.

13. Students Should Be Able To Adjust Clothing For Proper Fit.
Performance Indicators

    A.   Adjust straps.
    B.   Adjust belts.

14. Students Should Be Able To Put On Accessories Properly.
Performance Indicators

    A.   Put on gloves.
    B.   Put on hats.
    C.   Put on scarves.
    D.   Put on neck chains.
    E.   Put on bracelets.
    F.   Put on rings.
    G.   Put on earrings (if appropriate).
    H.   Put on watch.

15. Students Should Be Able To Choose Clothing Properly.
Performance Indicators

    A.   Choose clothing that coordinates.
    B.   Choose clothing appropriate for the weather.
    C.   Choose clothing appropriate for work.
    D.   Choose clothing appropriate for special events.
    E.   Choose clothing appropriate for play.

16. Students Should Be Able To Demonstrate Appropriate Clothing Care.
Performance Indicators

Levels:
I   A.   Puts dirty clothes in laundry container.
       B.   Hangs up clean clothes.
       C.   Puts clean clothes in drawer.
II.   D.   Cleans and polishes shoes.
       E.   Replaces worn shoe laces.
       F.   Sews on missing buttons.
III.   G.   Mends torn clothing by hand sewing.
       H.   Mends torn clothing using sewing machine.
       I.   Mends torn clothing with iron on patches.
       J.   Takes nonwashable clothing to cleaners.
       K.   Stores seasonal clothes appropriately when not in use.

17. Students Should Be Able To Demonstrate How To Use A Laundry Area
Performance Indicators

Levels:
I   A. Loads clothing into washing machine.
      B. Puts detergent into washer.
      C. Starts washer.
      D. Transfers items from washer to dryer.
      E. Starts dryer.
      F. Removes clothing from dryer.
      G. Hangs clothes on clothesline or rack.
II   H. Identifies soiled clothing.
      I. Sorts light from dark colored clothing.
      J. Measures detergent.
      K. Recognizes when clothes are dry.
      L. Cleans dryer filter.
      M. Folds clothes.
      N. Hangs clothes.
III O. Sorts clothes by fabric (delicate, permanent press, etc.).
      P. Selects correct washer and dryer settings for various materials and colors.
      Q. Uses powdered/liquid bleach appropriately.
      R. Uses spot remover appropriately.
      S. Identifies size of wash load.
      T. Selects and washes by hand hand-washable clothing.

18. Students Should Be Able To Clean a Bathroom.

Performance Indicators

Levels:
I   A. Clean a bathroom counter and sink.
      B. Empty wastebaskets.
      C. Sweep floors.
      D. Knock on closed bathroom door before entering.
II   E. Mop floors.
      F. Vacuum floors.
      G. Clean windows/mirrors.
      H. Clean a bathroom shower.
      I. Clean a bathtub.
      J. Hang clean towels and washclothes.
III K. Clean a toilet.
      L. Keep drains clear.
      M. Unclog toilet or sink with plunger.
      N. Recognize when bathroom needs to be cleaned.
      O. Replace bathroom supplies when needed.
      P. Return cleaning materials to correct storage area.

19. Students Should Be Able To Clean a Living/Dining Area

Performance Indicators

Levels:
I   A. Clear the floor.
      B. Empty ashtrays.
      C. Dust furniture.

II	D.	Sweep floors.
	E.	Vacuum carpet and floors.
III	F.	Care for rugs.
	G.	Wax floors.
	H.	Polish furniture.
	I.	Shampoo carpet.
	J.	Recognize when living/dining area needs to be cleaned.

20. Students Should Be Able To Demonstrate How To Clean a Bedroom

Performance Indicators

Levels:

I	A.	Pick up and put away belongings.
	B.	Empty wastebaskets.
	C.	Dust furniture surfaces.
	D.	Make a bed.
II	E.	Sweep the floor.
	F.	Vacuum the floor.
	G.	Change the bed.
III	H.	Clean mirrors and windows.
	I.	Clean closet.

21. Students Should Be Able To Demonstrate the Ability To Clean a Kitchen

Performance Indicators

Levels:

I	A.	Sweep the floor.
	B.	Wipe the counters.
	C.	Empty the garbage.
	D.	Wash and rinse dishes by hand.
	E.	Dry dishes.
	F.	Put dishes away.
II	G.	Clean major appliance surfaces.
	H.	Wash windows.
	I.	Wash walls.
	J.	Mop the floor.
	K.	Clean the sink.
	L.	Wipe small appliances clean.
III	M.	Identify household cleaning equipment.
	N.	Clean a freezer.
	O.	Clean an oven.
	P.	Wax a floor.
	Q.	Use checklist for cleaning a kitchen.
	R.	Clean inside of refrigerator.

22. Students Should Be Able To Demonstrate Knowledge of Safety Procedures In the Kitchen

Performance Indicators

Levels:
I   A.   Clean up debris of spills.
    B.   Do not touch a hot stove.
II C.   Wash knives by themselves.
    D.   Use small knife for peeling.
    E.   Use broom and dustpan for sweeping up broken objects.
    F.   Use pot holder.
    G.   Avoid putting knife or fork into a toaster.
    H.   Use electric appliances with dry hands.
III I.   Unplug cords safely.
    J.   Avoid overcrowding outlets.
    K.   Demonstrate knowledge of fire procedures.
    L.   Demonstrate knowledge of summoning help when needed.
    M.   Use matches safely.

23. Students Should Be Able To Demonstrate Meal Preparation Skills
Performance Indicators
Levels:
I   A.   Prepares simple drink.
    B.   Prepares simple snack.
II C.   Prepares simple breakfast with no cooking following picture recipe.
    D.   Prepares simple lunch with no cooking following picture recipe.
    E.   Prepares simple dinner with no cooking following picture recipe.
    F.   Prepares snack with no cooking following picture recipe.
III G.   Prepares simple breakfast requiring cooking following picture recipe.
    H.   Prepares simple lunch requiring cooking following picture recipe.
    I.   Prepares simple dinner requiring cooking following picture recipe.
    J.   Prepares snack with cooking following picture recipe.
IV K.   Follows a written recipe.
    L.   Demonstrates common food preparation tasks.
    M.   Plans meals for entire day.
V   N.   Plans meals for entire week.
    O.   Prepares advanced level meal (using skills in Objective L).

24. Students Should Be Able To Set the Table Correctly
Performance Indicators
Levels:
I   A.   Set the table using a marked placement.
II B.   Set the table using an unmarked placement.
III C.   Set the table using the chair as a visual cue.
    D.   Set the table correctly for a family of four.

25. Students Should Be Able To Demonstrate Meal Serving Skills
Performance Indicators
Levels:

I	A.	Serve themselves (drink and cereal).
	B.	Pass to next person.
II	C.	Serve themselves with little or no spills.
	D.	Pass to specific person.
	E.	Demonstrate knowledge of serving utensils: pitcher, large serving spoon and fork.
	F.	Take one from a platter and pass the rest on.
III	G.	Locate appropriate serving dishes.
	H.	Place dish on counter.
	I.	Locate pot of food.
	J.	Pour off excess liquid.
	K.	Locate and choose utensils.
	L.	Pour content of pot into dish without spilling.
	M.	Wipe up any spills on counter or serving dish.
	N.	Locate clean serving utensil.
	O.	Place dish and utensil on table.

26. Students Should Be Able To Demonstrate Ability To Clear Table
Performance Indicators
Levels:

I	A.	Remove serving dishes from table.
	B.	Scrape garbage from dishes.
II	C.	Rinse dishes.
	D.	Stack dishes.
	E.	Place utensils in dishpan or sink.
III	F.	Wipe table.
	G.	Store sponge properly.
	H.	Store leftover food in small air tight container or wrap with wrapping material and place in correct storage.

27. Students Should Demonstrate the Ability To Operate Home Equipment
Performance Indicators
Levels:

I	A.	Turn light switch on and off.
	B.	Place lids on pots and pans.
	C.	Operate flashlight on and off.
	D.	Turn knobs on doors.
	E.	Open/close twist-off bottle cap.
II	F.	Insert plugs into electrical outlets.
	G.	Lock/unlock door inside the house.
	H.	Hook/unhook latch.
	I.	Operate a safety chain on a door.
	J.	Operate electric fan.

K. Unlock door with a key.
L. Unlock lock with a key.
III. M. Operate a push-button phone.
N. Operate a dial phone.
O. Adjust thermostats.
P. Operate a window air conditioner.
Q. Operate a combination lock.
R. Replace light bulbs.

26. Students Should Be Able To Demonstrate Yard Care Skills
Performance Indicators
Levels:
I A. Waters yard/plants.
B. Keeps yard/sidewalks/driveways clear of obstacles and trash.
C. Appropriately disposes of garbage.
II D. Pulls weeds.
E. Plants flowers, bushes, trees.
F. Rakes a yard.
G. Operates a hand lawn mower.
III H. Trims grass edges.
I. Operates a power lawn mower.
J. Trims trees/bushes.
K. Fertilizes a yard.

State of the Art Resources

Effective instructional programs within the domestic living skills domain will be enhanced by knowledge of existing programs that contain successful teaching strategies. Residential staff members should have access to a word processor where a complilation of successful instructional programs can be retrieved in selected skill areas within the domestic domain. By coding each entry (i.e., EP=emergency phone calls, SM=self medication), articles can be retrieved in a category and trainers can have access to current state of the art procedures. The following section contains an initial list of articles that these authors feel contribute to an initial data bank of available domestic living skills programs from several journals in the field of special education.

Domestic Skills Instruction

AI = Academic Instruction
CM = Communication

CO =   Cooking
DC =   Domestic Chore
DR =   Dressing
EP =   Emergency Phone Calls
ES =   Emergency Skills, General
FE =   Feeding
GE =   General
IG =   Instruction, General
ME =   Mending
MO =   Mobility
OH =   Oral Hygiene
PU =   Punishment
SC =   Self-Care
SM =   Self-Medication
SS =   Social Skills
TO =   Toileting
WC =   Weight Control

Partial Source List of
Available Domestic Living Skill Programs

Adelson-Bernstein, N., & Wandow, L. (1978). Teaching buttoning to severely/profoundly retarded multihandicapped children. *Education and Training of the Mentally Retarded, 13,* 178-183.
DR
SC

Alberto, P., Jobes, N., Sizemore, A., & Doran, D.A. (1980). Comparison of individual and group instruction across response tasks. *Journal of the Association for the Severely Handicapped, 5,* 285-293.
IG

Albin, J.B. (1977). Some variables influencing the maintenance of acquired self-feeding behavior in profoundly retarded children. *Mental Retardation, 15*(5), 49-52.
FE

Bacon-Prue, A., Blout, R., Hosey, C., & Drabman, R. S. (1980). The public posting of photographs as a reinforcer for bedmaking in an institutional setting. *Behavior Therapy, 11,* 417-420.
DC

Banerdt, B., & Bricker, D. (1977). A training program for selected self-feeding skills for motorically impaired. *AAESPH Review, 3,* 222-229.
FE

Bauman, K. E., & Iwata, B.A. (1977). Maintenance of independent house-keeping skills using scheduling plus self-recording procedures. *Behavior Therapy, 8,* 554-560.
DC

Brickey, M. (1978). A behavioral procedure for teaching self-medication. *Mental Retardation, 16,* 29-32.
SC
SM

Carey, R. G., & Bucher, B. (1981). Identifying the educative and suppressive effects of positive practice and restitutional overcorrection. *Journal of Applied Behavior Analysis, 14,* 71-80. (using eating examples)
PU

Carroll, S. W., Sloop, E. W., Mutter, S., & Prince, P. L. (1976). The elimination of chronic clothes ripping in retarded people through a combination of procedures. *Mental Retardation, 1976, 16,* 246-249.
DR
PU

Close, D. W. (1977). Community living for severely and profoundly retarded adults: A group home study. *Education and Training of the Mentally Retarded, 12,* 256-262.
GE

Courtnage, L., Stainback, W., & Stainback, S. (1982). Managing prescription drugs in school. *Teaching Exceptional Children, 15*(1), 5-9.
SM

Crnic, K. A., & Pym, H. A. (1979). Training mentally retarded adults in independent living skills. *Mental Retardation, 17,* 13-16.
IG

Cronin, K. A., & Cuvo, A. J. (1979). Teaching mending skills to mentally retarded adolescents. *Journal of Applied Behavior Analysis, 12,* 401-406.
DC
ME

Cuvo, A. J., Jacobi, L., & Sipko, R. (1981). Teaching laundry skills to mentally retarded students. *Education and Training of the Mentally Retarded, 16,* 54-64.
DC

Doleys, D. M., Stacy, D., & Knowles, S. (1981). Modification of grooming behavior in adult retarded: Token reinforcement in a community-based program. *Behavior Modification, 5,* 119-128.
SC

Durana, I. L., & Cuvo, A. J. (1980). A comparison of procedures for decreasing public disrobing of an institutionalized profoundly mentally retarded woman. *Mental Retardation, 18,* 185-188.
DR
PU

Edgar, E., Maser, J., Smith, D. D., & Haring, N. G. (1977). Developing an instructional sequence for teaching a self-help skill. *Education and Training of the Mentally Retarded, 12,* 42-51.
IG

Fowler, S. A., Johnson, M. R., Whiteman, T. L., & Zukotynski, G. (1977).

Teaching a parent in the home to train self-help skills and increase compliance in her profoundly retarded adult daughter. *AAESPH Review,* 3, 151-161.
SC

Foxx, R. M. (1976). The use of overcorrection to eliminate the public disrobing (stripping) of retarded women. *Behaviour Research and Therapy,* 14, 53-61.
PU

Freagon, S., & Rotatori, A. F. (1982). Comparing natural and artificial environments in teaching self-care skills to group home residents. *The Journal of The Association for the Severely Handicapped,* 1982, 7(3), 73-86.
SC

Freagon, S., Wheeler, J., Hill, L. Brankin, G., & Costello, D. (1982), November). A domestic training environment for severely handicapped students. Unpublished manuscript presented for a poster session at the annual convention of The Association for the Severely Handicapped (TASH).
GE

Gruber, B., Reeser, R., & Reid, D. H. (1979). Providing a less restrictive environment for profoundly retarded persons by teaching independent walking skills. *Journal of Applied Behavior Analysis,* 12, 285-297.
MO

Halle, J. W., Marshall, A. M., & Spradlin, J. E. (1979). Time delay: A technique to increase language use and facilitate generalization in retarded children. *Journal of Applied Behavior Analysis,* 12, 431-439.
CM
IG

Hamre-Nietupski, S., & Williams, W. (1977). Implementation of selected sex education and social skills to severely handicapped students. *Education and Training of the Mentally Retarded,* 1977, 12, 364-372.
SS

Horner, R. D., & Keilitz, I. (1975). Training mentally retarded adolescents to brush their teeth. *Journal of Applied Behavior Analysis,* 8, 301-309.
OH

Johnson, B. F., & Cuvo, A. J. (1981). Teaching mentally retarded adults to cook. *Behavior Modification,* 5, 187-202.
CO

Jones, R. T., & Kazdin, A. E. (1980). Teaching children how and when to make emergency telephone calls. *Behavior Therapy,* 11, 509-521.
EP

Jones, R. T., Kazdin, A. E., & Haney, B. T. A follow-up to training emergency skills. *Behavior Therapy,* 12, 716-722.

Jones, R. T., Kazdin, A. E., & Haney, J. I. (1981). Social validation and training of emergency fire safety skills for potential injury prevention and life saving. *Journal of Applied Behavior Analysis,* 14, 249-260.

ES

Kissel, R. C., Johnson, M. R., & Whitman, T. L. (1980). Training a retarded client's mother and teacher through sequenced instructions to establish self-feeding. *Journal of the Association for the Severely Handicapped, 5,* 382-392.

FE

Kramer, L., & Whitehurst, C. (1981). Effects of button features on self-dressing in young retarded children. *Education and Training of the Mentally Retarded, 16,* 277-283.

DR

Lancioni, G. E. (1980). Teaching independent toileting to profoundly retarded deaf-blind children. *Behavior Therapy, 11,* 234-249.

TO

Leff, R. B. (1975) *How to use the telephone.* Paoli, PA: The Instructo Corporation.

EP

Matson, J. L. (1980). Preventing home accidents: A training program for the retarded. *Behavior Modification, 4,* 397-410.

ES

Matson, J. L., Marchetti, A., Adkins, J. A. (1980). Comparison of operant- and independent-training procedures for mentally retarded adults. *American Journal of Mental Deficiency, 84,* 487-494.

IG

Mitchell, L., Doctor, R. M., & Butler, D. C. (1978). Attitudes of caretakers toward the sexual behavior of mentally retarded persons. *American Journal of Mental Deficiency, 83, 289-296.*

SS

Murray, J. A., & Epstein. L.H. (1981). Improving oral hygiene with videotape modeling. *Behavior Modification, 5, 360-371.*

OH

Nutter, D., & Reid, D. H. (1978). Teaching retarded women a clothing selection skill using community norms. *Journal of Applied Behavior Analysis, 11,* 475-487.

DR

O'Brien, F., Bugle, C., & Arzin, N. H. (1972). Training and maintaining a retarded child's proper eating. *Journal of Applied Behavior Analysis, 5,* 67-72.

FE

Owings, N. O., & McManus, M. D. (1980). An analysis of communication functions in the speech of a deinstitutionalized adult mentally retarded client. *Mental Retardation, 18,* 309-314.

CM

Richman, J. S., Sonderby, T., Kahn, J. V. (1980). Prerequisites vs. in vivo acquisition of self-feeding skill. *Behavior Research and Therapy, 18,* 327-332.

FE

Risley, R., & Cuvo, A. J. (1980). Training mentally retarded adults to make emergency telephone calls. *Behavior Modification, 4,* 513-525.

EP
Robinson-Wilson, M. A. (1977). Picture recipe cards as an approach to teaching severely and profoundly retarded adults to cook. *Education and Training of the Mentally Retarded, 12,* 69-73.
CO
Rotatori, A. F., & Fox, R. (1980). The effectiveness of a behavioral weight reduction program for moderately retarded adolescents. *Behavior Therapy, 11,* 410-416.
WC
Rotatori, A. F., Fox, R., & Switzky, H. (1980). A multicomponent behavioral program for achieving weight loss in the adult mentally retarded person. *Mental Retardation, 18,* 31-33.
WC
Schleien, S. J., Ash, T., Kiernan, J., & Wehman, P. (1981). Developing independent cooking skills in a profoundly retarded woman. *The Journal of the Association for the Severely Handicapped, 6*(2), 23-29.
CO
Sigelman, C., Ater, C., & Spanhel, C. (1976). Sex-role stereotypes and the homemaking participation of mentally retarded people. *Mental Retardation, 16,* 357-358.
DC
Smith, M., & Meyers, A. (1979). Telephone-skills training for retarded adults: Group and individual demonstrations with and without verbal instruction. *American Journal of Mental Deficiency, 83,* 581-587.
EP
Smith, P. S. (1979). A comparison of different methods of toilet training in the mentally handicapped. *Behaviour Research and Therapy, 17,* 33-43.
TO
Spears, D. L., Rusch, F. R., York, R., & Lilly, M. S. (1981). Training independent arrival behaviors to a severely mentally retarded child. *The Journal of the Association for the Severely Handicapped, 6*(2), 40-45.
MO
Swain, J. J., Allard, G. B. & Holborn, S. W. (1982). The good toothbrushing game: A school-based dental hygiene program for increasing the toothbrushing effectiveness of children. *Journal of Applied Behavior Analysis, 15,* 171-176.
OH
Thinesen, P. J., & Bryan, A. J. (1981). The use of sequential pictoral cues in the initiation and maintenance of grooming behaviors with mentally retarded adults. *Mental Retardation, 19,* 246-250.
SC
Thompson, T. J. Braam, S. J., & Fugua, R. W. (1982). Training and generalization of laundry skills: A multiple probe evaluation with handicapped persons. *Journal of Applied Behavior Analysis, 15,* 177-182.
DC

Thurlow, M. L., & Turnure, J. E. (1977). Children's knowledge of time and money: Effectiveness instruction for the mentally retarded. *Education and Training of the Mentally Retarded, 12,* 203-232.
AI

Tucker, D. J., & Berry, G. W. (1980). Teaching severely multihandicapped students to put on their own hearing aids. *Journal of Applied Behavior Analysis, 13,* 65-75.
SC

VanBiervliet, A., Spangler, P. F., & Marshall, A. M. (1981). An ecobehavioral examination of a simple strategy for increasing mealtime language in residential facilities. *Journal of Applied Behavior Analysis, 14,* 295-305.
CM
FE

Vlavell, J. E., McGimsey, J. F., & Jones, M. L. (1980). Rapid eating in the retarded: Reduction by nonaversive procedures. *Behavior Modification, 4,* 481-492.
FE

Vogelsberg, R. T., Anderson, J., Berger, P., Haselden, T., Mitwell, S., Schmidt, C., Skowron, A., Ulett, D., & Wilcox, B. (1980). Programming for apartment living: A description and rationale of an independent living skills inventory. *Journal of the Association for the Severely Handicapped, 5,* 38-54.
GE

Walls, R. T., Crist, K., Sienicki, D. A., & Brant, L. (1981). Prompting sequences in teaching independent living skills. *Mental Retardation, 19,* 242-245.
IG

Wambold, C., & Salisbury, C. (1977). The development and implementation of self-care programs with severely and profoundly handicapped children. *AAESPH Review, 3,* 178-184.
SC

Willette, J. C., & Savage, J. A. (1978). Positive motivation: A method for promoting oral health among mentally retarded people. *Mental Retardation, 16,* 233-235.
OH

Williams, Jr., F. E., & Sloop, E. W. (1978). Success with a shortened Foxx-Azrin toilet training program. *Education and Training of the Mentally Retarded, 13,* 399-402.
TO

Chapter 9

Leisure Time Activities

THE PLEASURABLE and efficient use of leisure time can be a significant measure of successful living. The appropriate use of these time periods may have little to do with an individual's financial or social status. The numerous activities that are possible for one to enjoy in their leisure time is often a reflection of one's education.

Individuals who have received appropriate education and training in leisure time activities can realize continual benefits in their personal leisure time pursuits. Time away from school, workshop or other vocational endeavors includes pursuit of personal interest in activities, hobbies or recreational undertakings.

By contrast, however, individuals who have time on their hands and nothing to do (dead time) fail to participate in enjoyable pursuits. Excessive sitting, wandering or viewing television allow for little benefit mentally, physically, emotionally, or socially. Continuous waste of such leisure opportunities by an individual can certainly detract from defining a quality of life.

The seriousness of leisure time waste for individuals who are handicapped surfaced recently when the authors conducted research in leisure time activities. The participants in the study were adults who worked at a sheltered workshop. A questionnaire asked parents of these individuals how their son or daughter occupied their leisure time. A frequency of responses for the two items follows:

a) Do you feel that your son or daughter uses his/her leisure time adequately?

65	68
Yes	No

b) If your answer to number a is *no*, what reasons can you give for this?
(check as many as necessary)
#35 a) needs to know more leisure time activities
#16 b) needs games and equipment for leisure time
#44 c) needs other people to play with
9 d) other reasons (please list)

It is interesting to note that the above survey contained information that over half of the parents responding felt that their son or daughter did not utilize their leisure time adequately. Although a high percentage of parents answered this question in the negative, this figure could conceivably be higher due to parental protectiveness, feeling they would be considered inadequate parents if they were poor providers of leisure time activities for their son/daughter. Also, one must consider the parental definition of adequate leisure time: parents may have felt that excessive television watching is an appropriate leisure time activity.

Research question b, concerning reasons given for inadequate leisure time, emphasizes two important points: these handicapped adults needed to be involved more with other individuals in their leisure time activities and that they needed more educational training in this area. Figure 9.1 contains all items of the questionnaire.

Many investigators of leisure activities for moderately retarded adolescents suggest that most of these individuals occupy a great deal of their time watching television. Also, Madison Metropolitan School District in a follow-up study of moderately and severely retarded graduates of their program found that parents and guardians of these individuals felt that following graduation these retarded individuals experienced extremely limited leisure time and recreational opportunities.

Even without any objective research findings concerning handicapped individuals and their use of leisure time, personal observations seem to continuously reaffirm that handicapped individuals, as a group, use their leisure time in an inadequate manner. This inadequate utilization of time can be contributed, in most instances, to nonexistent leisure time training programs. For example, in the area of leisure time activities in residential homes, a staff member that turns on the television set every night for the home's leisure time activity is performing a disservice for the residents. The disservice involves the staff member's omission of an educational program for the residents in the area of alternative leisure time activities available for each resident. Life involves choices, but one must be aware of the choices available. Residents often are not aware of the leisure time opportunities available to them.

This chapter provides direction for residential staff in providing leisure time programming. The commitment of a residential facility to a structured leisure educational program for its residents is a vital one.

Fig. 9.1 **Leisure Time Questionaire**

1. Do you feel that your son or daughter uses their leisure time adequately? (Check one). Yes ☐   No ☐
COMMENT:

2. If your answer to number 1 is *no,* what reasons can you give for this? (Check as many as necessary.)
☐ (a) needs to know more leisure time activities
☐ (b) needs games and equipment for leisure time
☐ (c) needs other people to play with
☐ (d) other reasons (please list)

3. Do you feel your son or daughter watches too much television:
Yes ☐ No ☐
COMMENT:

Estimated hours per week _____ ?

4. Do you feel your son or daughter spends too much time listening to the radio or the record player?
Yes ☐ No ☐
COMMENT:

Estimated hours per week _____ ?

5. Would you *list* leisure time games or equipment that you have at home. (Examples: baseball, puzzles, cards, etc.)

6. What are your sons or daughters favorite leisure time activities?

7. Does your son or daughter enjoy spending their leisure time in: (Check one.)
outside activities ☐   indoor activities ☐

8. Does your son or daughter enjoy spending leisure time in quiet activities such as coloring or more physical activities such as running? (Check one.)

quiet activities ☐   physical activities ☐

9. If there are other children in the family, do they participate with your son or daughter in leisure time activities? (Check one.)

a great deal of time ☐   a little amount of time ☐

10. Would you check the following activities that your son or daughter participates in and list the approximate time per week spent in this activity? (Check as many as necessary and estimate time for each.)

Activity

Badminton

Tetherball

Ball Hitting—
   Softball

List additional activities

11. Would you list different activities that your family does with your son or daughter as a family group? (Check as many as necessary.)

☐ (a) Camping
☐ (b) Picnics
☐ (c) Drive-ins or movie shows
☐ (d) Family rides (other than business)
☐ (e) Going out to dinner
☐ (f) Other activities: please list

Estimate hours per week spent in such activities as a family group _____ .

List additional activities

Overview/Suggestions for Leisure Time Programming

General suggestions for a residential facility's leisure activity program follow. A genuine commitment is needed to develop and sustain an ongoing program. This commitment includes the entire staff from the residential director to the direct care workers.

A. Develop a Facility Philosophy Concerning Leisure Time Activities

There needs to be a total awareness by all individuals associated with the facility that leisure time programming is a continuous ongoing objective of the facility. Such a commitment should be reflected as a part of the written goals of the facility and denoted within job responsibilities when hiring new staff. Also residents' I.H.P.'s (Individual Habilitative Plans) should include a programmatic decision concerning each resident's leisure time program.

B. Hire a Programmer (Coordinator of Leisure Time Activities)

The decision by the facility administration to spend money for a full-time coordinator of leisure time activities will be money well spent. A decision to hire a part-time coordinator would only be advisable when the number of residents in the facility is quite small or the severity of the residents' handicapping conditions is so limited as to restrict the need for a full-time programmer. The leisure time programmer's job responsibility would be to insure that the commitment of the facility to the improvement of the residents' use of their leisure time is realized.

C. Offer the Program on a Consistent Basis

A leisure time activities program involving a residential facility for the handicapped must be offered to its residents on a consistent schedule to be effective. The consistent offering of a leisure time program is important for the following reasons:

a) Residents' interest in most activities occur when they are exposed to experiences on a regular basis so that ample time to learn and enjoy leisure time experiences is possible.
b) Residents can anticipate, plan and prepare themselves for leisure time experiences.

c) Residents can learn to suggest future leisure time activities that they would like to participate in.
d) Residents learn that during specific time periods they will be expected to participate in leisure time activities and that their participation is valued.

D. Know Your Residents

Individuals involved with leisure time programming need to continuously evaluate the residents in the facility to assess individual capabilities for participating in specific leisure time activities. The broad aspects of a comprehensive leisure activity program dictates each resident's abilities be considered. In this way matching residents' abilities to satisfying and rewarding experiences will help insure participation in a successful leisure time program.

E. Offer a Broad-Based Leisure Time Program

There are a vast number of leisure time activities that can be offered in most residential facilities. Sound programming entails a variety of leisure time activities. By providing a variety of activities, residents are given the opportunity to participate in a wide assortment of physical, sensory, and emotional experiences. Leisure time activities for residents promote their personal growth by broadening experiential opportunities.

F. Task Analyze the Leisure Time Activities

Task analysis refers to the division of a leisure activity into smaller components and teaching these components in a logical sequence. The use of task analyses is an important process for leisure programmers. Each leisure activity can be divided into more teachable steps that enables a resident to learn the task in a more efficient manner.

G. Allow Free Time Away from Any Structured Leisure Time Programming

Care must be exhibited in that the residents are allowed free time on their own to pursue their personal forms of interest and relaxation. The structured leisure time program must not become so overwhelming that it doesn't allow the residents time for themselves. Not everyone has to be busy all the time; one of the many pleasures of living in your own home is at times to just lean back and let the world go by. There needs to be, therefore, a sensible balance between formalized leisure time pursuits and a time that the residents can have for their own personal use.

H. Learn to Adapt the Leisure Time Activities to the Particular Needs of Your Residents

The ability to adapt leisure time activities to the special needs of your particular residents is an invaluable technique for any coordinator. Many leisure time activities have been created or developed for individuals who have average or above mental, physical, sensory, emotional and social ability. When using such leisure time activities with residents who have specific disabilities in certain of these areas, adjustments in adapting the leisure time activities must be made.

Many popular leisure time activities do not have to be eliminated from residential facility consideration if an adaptive version of the activity is still quite pleasurable and enjoyable for the residents. Lawn croquet, for example, can be especially adapted for a special group by increasing the size of the wickets, increasing the mallet head size, shortening the course, and allowing for numerous hits of the ball. Other adaptations may also be deemed necessary; if so, adapt. This will allow residents to enjoy specific specific leisure time activities that are commonly participated in by active members of society. Figure 9.2 contains an illustration of the building blocks that were described in the preceeding sections.

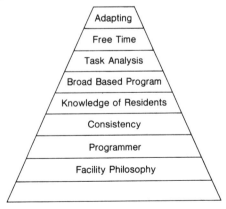

Fig. 9.2

Leisure Time Activity Content Areas

The wide spectrum of leisure time activities that are possible for inclusion in a comprehensive residential program can't possibly be covered in any one chapter. This section, however, will present certain leisure time program areas with suggestions of specific activities offered under each area. A leisure time activity coordinator will never find a complete list of leisure time activities, but should explore all possible reference material available, as well as continuously search for new activities operative in the active environment. The following listing will assist a leisure time activity coordinator in beginning this search.

Arts/Crafts:

Arts and crafts provide the participant with activities that use their manipulative skills to create and/or construct physical objects.

Art/Craft Activities: (sample listing)

Bead construction	Etching
Block printing	Finger painting
Burlap crafts	Flower making
Candle making	Gift wrapping
Cardboard construction	Knitting
Carving objects	Leather craft
Ceramics	Model building
Charcoal drawing	Mosaics
Clay modeling	Oil painting
Costume jewelry	Paper-mache crafts
Crayon drawing	Photography
Crepe paper craft	Plaster of paris
Crocheting	Pottery
Dressmaking	Quilting
Embroidery	Wood Crafts

Games/Table:

Table games provide the participant with activities that cover a wide variety of basically fun experiences that can be enjoyed around a table by oneself, another person, a small group or even at times a large number of people.

Games: (sample listing)

Avalanche	Jacks
Battleship	Labyrinth
Bean Bag Throw	Michigan Rummy
Bingo	Pick-Up-Sticks
Booby Trap	Pin Ball Type Games
Bowling (carpet)	Rack-O
Card (games)	Shuffleboard (table)
Checkers	Skittle Ball
Chinese Checkers	Sports Games (table)
Coloring games	Stadium Checkers
Cootie	Tiddly Winks
Dominoes	

Physical Fitness Activities:

Physical fitness activities provide the participant the opportunity for developing, improving and maintaining general health, personal strength, endurance and overall physical condition.

Physical Fitness Activities: (sample listing)

Body mechanics	Jogging
Calisthenics	Obstacle courses
Circuit exercise training	Relays
Fitness testing	Running
Interval training	Walking
Jazz-O-Cise (exercises)	Weight training

Hobbies:

Hobbies provide the participant with a number of highly interesting activities than can be pursued on a personal level during one's leisure time moments.

Hobbies: (sample listing)

Aquariums	Gardening
Baking (e.g. cookies)	Plants (indoor, outdoor)
Bird watching	Raising pets
Collections (e.g. baseball cards)	Refinishing furniture
	Wood building (e.g. flower boxes)

Sports/Games:

Sports/games provide the participant with many different group games that foster cooperative team play, sound physical development and healthy exercise.

Sports/Games: (sample listing)

Badminton	Shuffleboard
Basketball	Soccer
Bowling	Softball
Croquet	Table Tennis
Horseshoes	Tetherball
Paddle Tennis	Volleyball

Social Activities:

Social activities provide the participants with a specific interaction with other individuals that fosters friendships and a personal warmth developed from being an integral part of a group of people.

Social Activities: (sample listing)

Barbecues	Marshmallow roasts
Birthday parties	Picnics
Church socials	Potluck suppers
Clubs	Scavenger hunts
Costume parties	Soda pop parties
Dances	Suppers
Eating out	Treasure hunts
Holiday celebrations	Wiener roasts

The following section contains selected activities from each leisure time content area. It would be beyond the scope of this chapter to discuss each activity within each area, however, a discussion of some of these activities should be helpful.

Arts/Crafts

Clay Modeling:

A beneficial activity for those residents who have adequate

manipulative ability with their hands. This activity develops self-expression in that an individual is offered a great deal of latitude in the creation of a finished product. Such finished projects can cover the gamut from a purely abstract creation to a realistic representation of some environmental object.

Another benefit of clay modeling activities is the pure joy that so many individuals receive from the tactile manipulation of the clay material itself. Additionally, the finished product is a permanent object that can give one pleasure for years or that can be given away as a gift to friends. This permanence of an object, a real advantage, is true of most arts and crafts projects.

Model Building

Model crafts appeals to both males and females. The appeal of model building is that the finished product is a replica of some object that exists in the environment. Those individuals who enjoy model building delight in the replication of smaller but identifiable environment objects. The strict procedures necessary to complete a finished model will also attract certain residents who need a rather highly organized activity.

A real disadvantage to model building is that many of the model kits are quite complex and often require a high degree of eye-hand coordination. Selection of appropriate models for the resident is critical. Assistance from staff members should be available to assist residents in model building.

Photography

Thousands of individuals enjoy the leisure time activity of photography. The reason so many people find this hobby interesting is because photography helps us remember previous events. Many individuals with significant handicaps can develop into successful photographers. They can enjoy the beauty of photographs by themselves or share their work with their friends. There is such a wide range of photographic equipment available for almost anyone's budget to accomodate this hobby.

The challenge to the leisure time coordinator is the adaptations of the equipment for specific handicapping conditions. Definite challenges will exist in equipment adjustments, but camera shops, photography clubs and enthusiasts of this hobby will be more than willing to assist. Also, special care must be given so that complete and repeated instructions are given to those residents selecting such a leisure time hobby.

Games/Table

Bingo

The game of bingo is an activity that can be enjoyed by a few individuals or a large group. It's an excellent game for a residential home because many different varieties of bingo can be created so as to meet those special needs of the particular residents. For example, a bingo game could be created for residents with basic abilities using a board consisting of two different shapes or colors, whereas for residents with advanced abilities a board consisting of numerous words or sentences could be constructed.

Another nice feature of bingo as a leisure time activity is that inexpensive prizes can be offered as rewards for participation. Prizes can be offered for any form of leisure time participation, but with bingo it has always been an intricate part of the game. Also, bingo can be an advantage to those residents who have a short attention span because each draw can move at such a fast rate. It is good to remember also that bingo can be used to teach many concepts: numbers, colors, shapes, words, symbols and others. The coordinator has the responsibility to use imagination in the selection of such concepts and to make it practical and functional so that the residents are having fun and learning at the same time.

Sports Games (Table)

There are a multitude of different sports games on the market that can be played on a table top. These games cover a wide variety of sports and contain challenging skills necessary for participation. Many table games are quite exciting and a great deal of fun to play. The leisure time coordinator, however, must be careful to match the level of skill involved in each game to the particular residents of the home. To emphasize further, this leisure time activity is considerable fun but only when the sports games are at the resident's appropriate skill level; it is a costly inappropriate purchase when these sports games are too advanced for fun participation.

Physical Fitness

Calisthenics

The regular use of a vital calisthenics program for certified (physican approved) residents is a healthy undertaking. There are two important considerations to the success of an excercise program. The first consideration is that a program is offered on a regular basis—same time, same days. If the program is offered in a haphazard manner, residents will not improve their health and interest in activities will be diminished. The second consideration is that the calisthenics program should be vigorous enough for each individual, so that a certain amount of improvement can be realized by each resident. The program can be offered to a group but have individualized goals for each participant, goals that are a realistic challenge.

In discussion of this last point, individualization of the exercise program by documentation of each resident's progress on charts will help to challenge the resident towards further progress. This charting of each individual's accomplishments will, in a visual manner, assist the resident in understanding his progress and hopefully motivate him towards reaching his personal goals. For those residents who have motivation problems but still participate, special rewards should be offered for reaching specific goals. As an example, a female resident who loses fifteen pounds can shop and purchase a new dress for herself. One final note, if the resident has the ability to record their own progress, they should be responsible for this charting. If they do not have such skills, be sure and include them in some manner in the charting. For such a resident, helping to hold the pencil can be an involvement, and by doing this residents may gain a better understanding of their progress.

Walking/Jogging

The exercise phenomenon in the '70s and '80s has been jogging and walking for improved general health. Proponents of this form of exercise relate improvements in such physical attributes as leg strength, a stronger cardiovascular system, weight loss, and other health benefits. All of these claims seem to justify the enthusiasm and individual's involvement in these exercise activities and do appear as a step towards a healthy life. Those residents who are interested and could participate in a walking-jogging program should be encouraged to take part.

The approval, however, of a physician for each resident who participates in such a program is mandatory. A sound safety precaution, for any person responsible for vigorous activity programs, is to obtain medical release for each individual who will be involved in a strenuous physical program. Similarly, the coordinator should enlist assistance form any or all of the following: a physical therapist, occupational therapist, physical education director, recreational specialist, or other health experts.

The utilization of appropriate jogging equipment is essential to the success of such a program. Number one on this equipment list is appropriate running shoes. A vigorous walking or jogging program will place an individual's feet under tremendous stress and strain. The running shoe should be purchased with the particular physical and structure need of each resident in mind. Furthermore, walking and jogging clothing should be carefully selected for the appropriate seasonal changes, clothing that offers the resident the correct type of insulation and protection from fluctuating weather conditions. Careful examination of the equipment, clothing and protective devices necessary for a walking and/or jogging program is a necessary program standard.

Hobbies

Aquariums:

The hobby of establishing and maintaining an aquarium is a pleasurable use of leisure time. There has never been a more advantageous time for those individuals interested in aquariums. Speciality shops that sell aquarium products have a wide variety of supplies and a marvelous selection of fish for purchase. Whereas at one time, aquarium supplies and fish were quite expensive, this is no longer the situation, as prices now cover a wide range of purchasing options.

Those residents who would enjoy having their own aquarium should be taken to speciality shops and shown the available options. During the process of establishing and maintaining an aquarium, ensure that the resident takes on the necessary responsibilities that accompany this activity. The resident must have the ability to maintain the equipment and contribute to the eventual improvement of the aquarium.

Gardening

The rewards of participating in this hobby are many: exercise, fresh air, and the joy of nurturing growth. These are all admirable features of gardening and residents who possess the ability and desire to begin this activity should understand the process of seed growth. They will need to be shown pictures of the expected produce and if possible the actual product itself. At the same time and during the life of the garden, appropriate maintenance responsibilities must be emphasized and continuously demonstrated and monitored until residents are able and willing to maintain the garden. Gardening is a wonderful hobby and residents of residential facilities should be encouraged, when possible, to participate in such an activity.

Sports/Games

Bowling:

There are many different types of bowling events that can be devised. The most obvious form of bowling is that performed at your local bowling alley. The residential facility, however, can provide other opportunities that are fun and similar to the bowling alley version. The purchase of plastic bowling pins and a realistic plastic bowling ball is equipment that can be used to create a bowling alley in the recreation room or the basement of the residential facility. Also, bowling equipment that is of a more durable plastic or even wood can serve a similar purpose on the concrete driveway or even the facility's lawn. If the residents participate in a bowling alley's program on a regular basis, such residential practice would improve their competencies for this activity; if not, home participation is still a fun activity.

In discussing a regular bowling program for the residents, such a program should be seriously considered by the leisure time coordinator if the residents like such an activity and have the aptitude for the activity. The social benefits derived by the residents from a community based program are worthwhile. An evening part-icipating at the local bowling alley with other leagues comprised of community residents is a wonderful opportunity for the residents to be seen and known by the local community. There may be at times some problems associated with this involvement, especially initially as the community adjusts to the presence of the residents, but the long term involvement should be a triumph for community integration and along with this worthwhile benefit—bowling is a fun night out.

Volleyball

A good group activity is the game of volleyball. So often when passing a group outing we view an active game of volleyball taking place—children, young adults, adults and seniors participating in a pleasurable activity. Because volleyball is a good group activity, serious consideration should be given to including it in your residential leisure time activity program.

The important consideration in providing a volleyball program for a residential facility is the amount of adaptation necessary to meet specific needs of the residents. One of the real advantages of volleyball as an activity in a residential facility is that the game can be changed to meet many different ability levels. As examples, the net can be lowered, a larger, softer ball can be used, the ball may be caught and thrown back over the net, boundaries can be enlarged, and other variations of the proper rules or regulations of the game can be changed; all of these things and more can be done to accommodate different ability levels.

Social

Dances

Those residential facilities that have residents who chronologically and socially are mature enough to benefit from attending dances should be provided this opportunity. A dance situation provides a social gathering where residents can benefit in personal growth from atttending. Cleaning up to get ready, wearing the right clothes, practicing our best manners, and talking appropriately to others are a few examples of what an individual can learn from participating in a mixed social gathering like a dance.

In providing this leisure time activity be sure and use felxibility in the judgment of how each resident will respond to this type of activity. For some residents an event like a dance may be a very natural social situation, however, for other residents it may be a very awkward and frightening personal experience. The programmer must be aware of what to expect from each resident in attending this type of social function. Individual differences will certainly be apparent in those residents attending a dance, and flexibility in how we handle these different behaviors should reflect our understanding and allowances granted for each resident.

Picnics

Almost everyone enjoys going on a picnic. Picnics provide individuals with the opportunity to be outside, enjoy good food, be in the company of others, participate in games and activities and other outdoor experiences.

In planning for picnics, however, the coordinators must not perform all the preparational activities by themselves. The facility's residents, even those with minimal abilities, should be included in the planning process and in the food preparation and the equipment organizations. It is a disservice to our residents when we don't include them in the planning and the preparation for these types of activities. Planning sessions should be held with the residents and specific picnic responsibilities assigned to each resident participating in the outing. By including the residents in this process, picnics become more personalized and definitely more fun for each resident.

Summary Content Areas

There are many other activities that can be included in a leisure time activity program: aquatics, musical activities, attending special events, community volunteer work and other type activities. As there are activities and events in life, so are there leisure times possibilities. An inquisitive, explorative mind, therefore, is an important attribute for any leisure time coordinator to develop. A coordinator must be cognitive of the particular interest of the facility's residents and also keenly aware of the leisure time opportunities that are available to any one individual.

Sample Instructional Formats for Selected Leisure Activities

Included in the following sections are sample instructional formats for teaching five leisure activities: Bingo, Chinese Checkers, Sliding, Tetherball, and Frisbee.

Bingo

Number of Participants:	Two or more
Equipment Needed:	Bingo Game
Associated Facilities Needed:	Table and Chairs
Past Learning and Associated Skills Involved:	Recognition of numbers, finger dexterity, and eye-hand coordination.

Body Position: Sitting   Comments:

Step 1   To start with, make larger than normal bingo cards with large markers and have the student place the card in front of himself.

Step 2:   Explain the free space and have the student practice placing the marker on the free space.

Step 3:   Teach the student to draw a number and read.

3 If the students have not learned numbers, color or animal figures could be used.

Step 4   After the student has mastered drawing a number, show him how to cover the number on his card.

4 Use small numbers at first such as 1-5 or 1-10.

Step 5   After covering the numbers on the card is mastered, call the right numbers so the student practices getting bingo.

5 Be sure that it is understood that this is the object of the game.

Step 6   After the student can recognize a bingo in a straight line, explain a bingo across, etc.

Step 7   Now you can increase the number squares and size of both squares and markers to regulation.

Helpful Hints: If the student learns to draw and call the numbers it will make comprehending the game much easier; also the students will not have to depend on others to play the game.

Notes _____
_____
_____
_____

Chinese Checkers

Number of Participants:	Two through six
Equipment Needed:	Chinese checkers board and set
Associated Facilities Needed:	Tables and chairs
Past Learning and	
Associated Skills Involved:	Color distinction, finger dexterity, depth and visual perception, and eye-hand coordination.

Body Position: Sitting   Comments:

Step 1 Place the marble at the top of the triangle of the appropriate color.

           1 Start with one marble

Step 2 Next, teach the student to move the marble one space along the black line into the next hole.

Step 3 Convey the idea that the student is to move the marble along the black lines one move at a time until you have reached the triangle opposite the one you started.

           3 Some students will not go beyond this point, but to them moving the one marble may be a success, so don't get discouraged.

Step 4 Next, add another player with one marble, having the two move the marble each in turn to the opposite triangle.

Step 5 Have the students repeat Step 4 but this time arrange it so that their marbles come together. At this time teach them how to jump.

Step 6 After the foregoing group of steps is mastered, add another marble, teaching them to jump their own marbles and so on until they are using all the marbles. Add more players.

Helpful Hints: It may be easier for the students to start in an opposite color triangle going to the same color triangle as their marble. In the beginning a board may be made up with a straight line of holes; start a marble at each end to convey the idea of the game to lower ability students.

Notes _____

_____
_____

Slides

Number of Participants: One
Equipment Needed: Slide
Associates Facilities Needed: Area for the slide
Past Learning and
Associated Skills Involved: Body coordination, balance, eye-hand/
                                 eye-foot coordination.

Body Position: Standing, sitting   Comments:

Step 1 Student sits at the bottom
        of the slide.

Step 2 Demonstrate coming down   2 Stress safety at all times.
        the slide.

Step 3 Take the student around to   3 Begin with small slides.
        the ladder of the slide and
        grab hold of the railing
        with both hands.

Step 4 After student has both
        hands on the railing have him
        go up the first step and stop.

Step 5 After s/he has mastered the   5 Be sure that s/he does not fall
        first step, have him/her take   and give him/her confidence
        another step and so on until   by following him up.
        he is at the top.

Step 6 After reaching the top,   6 The teacher should go down
        have him/her sit down with   the slide with the student the
        his/her legs in the direction   first few times.
        of the slide.

Step 7 Have the student release
        his/her hold and proceed down
        the slide. Initially, if student shows
        fear, have him/her hold lightly
        onto the side of the slide.

Helpful Hints: By taking the ladder a step at a time, it will decrease any fear of height the student may have and help the student master the art of climbing a ladder. It may be necessary to go ahead of the student as well as having someone give support from behind in order for him to overcome his fear of the unknown. Small slides are available for classroom use.

Notes _____
_____
_____

Tetherball

Number of Participants:	One to four
Equipment Needed:	Pole, tetherball
Associated Facilities Needed:	Area in which to play
Past Learning and Associated Skills Involved:	Eye-hand coordination, visual and depth perception, reaction time, and body coordination and flexibility.

Body Position: Standing

Comments:

Step 1 Student learns to hit the ball with two hands in different directions.

1 It is important that the student keeps his eye on the ball.

Step 2 The student hits the ball with different amounts of power.

2 Initially, have student use two hands.

Step 3 One student can stand on each side of the pole and have a wall or object toward which he will hit the ball from the side of the pole.

Step 4 The student can hit the ball with either one hand or two and emphasis can be placed on wrapping the ball around the pole.

4 Introduce another player here—having both players trying to hit the ball and wrap the rope around the pole. Since the ball can be wrapped around the pole in two different directions, each player tries to wrap the ball around in an opposite direction in order to win.

Step 5 Four students can play the game with each student having one-fourth of the playing circle as his boundary and every other student being a partner.

Helpful Hints: A faster reaction time is the focus of attention in the latter stages of the sport. When the larger ball is mastered a smaller ball can be used with paddles for the more advanced students, adding more challenge to the game. Many skills invoved in this game are also involved in volleyball.

Notes _____

_____
_____

Frisbee

Number of Participants:	Two or more
Equipment Needed:	Flying saucer or Frisbee
Associated Facilities Needed:	Large open area
Past Learning and	
Associated Skills Involved:	Eye-hand coordination, body flexibility, visual perception, and depth perception

Body Position: Standing   Comments:

Step 1   Demonstrate how to hold the flying saucer, open part down and hand on the edge.

Step 2   Show how to sail it for a short distance at a large target.

1 If the student is elevated by standing at the top of steps it will make the initial throw easier and more reinforcing.

Step 3   Increase the distance and gradually decrease the size of the target.

Step 4   Have the student learn to catch the flying saucer.

4 In catching, it may be best to start with basket-catch or two hands.

Step 5   Have two people play catch at a short distance, increasing it as they get more proficient.

Step 6   Increase the number of participants.

Helpful Hints: Wind may be a factor in the control of the flying saucer. To make it easier for students just learning to throw, an enclosed space or a windless day is advised.

Notes _____

_____
_____

These developmental task forms are beginning steps for what could be developed into a more comprehensive task analysis of each leisure time activity. Although with certain residents these basic developmental steps would be quite adequate for instructional purposes, other residents will need a further task analysis of activities. To accomplish this objective, the leisure time coordinator will need to begin with the basic developmental steps for learning the activity and then use sound judgment concerning further analysis of the experience.

Partial Participation in an Activity

Although discussion in this chapter has dealt with the method and technique of adaptation in the instruction of leisure time activities, further emphasis is necessary. By adhering to a principle of partial participation, the coordinator adapts skills, sequence of movements, and materials to allow residents to enjoy activities that might not have been previously selected.

When making decisions about adapting an activity, there are questions that must be carefully answered:

1. Do the handicapped residents demonstrate an interest or desire to participate in the activity?
2. What parts of the activity are too difficult for the residents to participate in because of inappropriate skills and what skills do the residents have for adaptive participation?
3. How different will the adaptive version of the activity be from the actual activity itself?
4. After the activity has been adapted for the residents, is it still an enjoyable activity?
5. Is the activity one that residents can enjoy participation in for many months and years?
6. Does the adaptive version of the activity also allow participation and enjoyment of the activity by those residents who did not need a change in the original activity?
7. Is there special equipment that needs to be ordered or constructed so that the adaptive activity can be presented?
8. Has developmental instructional steps or a task analysis been developed for the actual instruction of the adaptive activity?

The development of adaptive skills in the organization of leisure activities demands creativity by recreation coordinators. Coordinators with leisure time responsibility must continuously challenge themselves for new ways in which individuals can participate in pleasurable leisure time pursuits. However, the challenge is worth the effort when one views the enjoyment of individuals now participating in an activity that before adaptation they could have only been involved in as spectators.

An example of adaptive methods for residents:

Softball
- not calling balls or strikes
- using the same capable pitcher for every batter
- shortening the bases
- going only to first and back home
- using a tee (stand) instead of a pitcher
- rolling a play ball (large) towards the batter
- laying a play ball (large) at home plate so the batter can hit
- hitting for certain players but letting these players move around the bases.

Residents with Restricted Leisure Time Abilities

There are residential facilities that have residents who are so severely involved that they can only be engaged in quite limited leisure time activities. These residents have extremely limited ability in some or all of the following: physical movement, mental capabilities, adequate behaviors and sensory acuity. These limitations create a difficult challenge to a leisure time coordinator planning meaningful activities for their participation.

In meeting this challenge, the leisure time programmer must think in terms of the process rather than in terms of the product. Process refers to experiences residents receive that are more important than waiting for a measurable behavioral result that may be exhibited. For example, a programmer placing a resident's hand into a pan of water and moving the hand up and down, splashing the water, running the hand along the bottom of the pan, across the top of the water and other like experiences with the water is creating an experience—a process. The objective is to provide the experience, create a process.

When offering leisure time experiences to residents with severe motor and sensory involvement, consider the following:

a) Include as many different forms of stimulation as possible—visual, auditory, tactile, kinesthetic, olfactory—make the experience multi-stimulating.

b) Strive for some behavioral response out of the resident.

c) Keep the experiences to a short time frame because of short attention spans, but repeat often, after resident has rested.

d) Involve as many different individuals as you can in offering such experiences; new people—new experience. (Train individuals in this type of programming.)

e) Change the sitting or lying position of the residents often, if possible; new position—new experience.

f) Create a circle arrangement when working with a number of residents; makes for ease of instruction and encourages more involvement by the residents.

Suggested Activities (sample)

These are some of the experiences that can be offered to the resident with restricted leisure time abilities. To use a variety of these experiences, however, a leisure time coordinator should be alert to new process type experiences that are present in the surrounding environment.

Record player	Tasting different foods
Water play	Drinking different liquids
Texture touching	Wearing different clothes
Smelling different scents	Rubbing different surfaces
Following objects with eyes	on the skin
Different noise makers	Assisted hand movements
Different body positions	Assisted leg movements
Riding things	Reaching for things
Swinging in things	Different basic music instruments

Community Involved Program

Whenever possible, residents should be involved in existing leisure time community programs. Along with actual participation in a leisure time activity, residents of the home will benefit tremendously from the social interaction with other individuals. This broader based leisure time community involvement will assist the residents to model more appropriate behaviors. Behaviors are more apt to occur that will facilitate their improved involvement in leisure time activities as well as a better understanding and utilization of proper social conduct.

A real effort should be made by the facility staff to include residents in an integrated community leisure time program. Local communities offer a wide variety of leisure time activities for their citizens. Facility personnel should carefully investigate these opportunities and seek out key individuals involved in these activities and solicit their assistance in including the residents in their programs. When seeking this assistance, keep in mind that resident participation can be at many different levels of involvement. For example, a resident may assist a local softball team as their equipment manager of if resident skills are adequate as a member of a community bowling team. This form of leisure time community integration is important, but will only occur if facility staff is willing to pursue this type of community involvement; it will take an effort.

A Final Thought

A residential facility must provide its residents with constructive, meaningful and pleasant leisure activities. Many of the residents lack direction, motivation or understanding of how to use their leisure time in an effective manner. To accomplish this objective, a leisure time coordinator must be employed.

This leisure time coordinator should accomplish two major objectives in such a program. The first objective is to disclose to the residents a variety of different leisure time activities that are possible for their active participation. And the second objective is to provide sound instruction in those activities so that resident can begin to enjoy their leisure time pursuits.

Chapter 10

General Community Functioning

A COMMON procedure many trainers use to enable residents to acquire functional community skills is to locate a task analysis from a published curriculum, evaluate residents using materials and equipment in the residence, and teach the activity with the systematic use of cue/correction procedures in combination with a reinforcement schedule. Although many residents subsequently learn many behaviors in this manner, it cannot be assumed that the general skill of that behavior has been acquired. In fact, a primary characteristic of residents with severe handicaps is their lack of generalization from a setting where a behavior has been acquired to settings where that behavior has not yet been taught. A commonly observed practice when a targeted behavior does not generalize to a new setting is to retrain the behavior in each new setting until the resident can perform the behavior in more and more environments. This strategy is referred to as sequential modification. An alternative strategy that more actively seeks to facilitate the generalization of behaviors from training to natural settings is developed in this chapter. Briefly, this alternative strategy requires that the training setting include as many common features as are found in the range of natural settings where the behaviors would normally occur. This strategy is referred to as "programming common stimuli." (Stokes and Baer, 1977)

Table 10.1 contains a seven step sequence to assist teachers in determining what training setting provides the most suitable environment to train a behavior and at the same time increase the probability of that behavior occurring in other untrained settings.

This step-by-step strategy will be illustrated using a handwashing activity.

Table 10.1 Seven Step Strategy for Enhancing the Generalization of _____ Activity

1. Interview resident, peers, and primary care providers to determine the frequency of contact with selected activity in all life functioning areas.
2. Locate specific environments where activities from step 1 occur.
3. Analyze characteristics of activities.
4. Develop data sheets to include a range of distinguishing features of activity sub-behaviors.
5. Use data sheets in environments of step 2.
6. Develop task analyses for the most frequently checked environments in step 1.
7. Develop training strategies.

Interview Resident, Peers, and Primary Care Providers

The purpose of this first step is to determine the amount of contact residents have with community environments. Specifically what is the frequency of participating in activities in domestic, vocational, recreation/leisure, and general community activities. Domestic settings could include a friend or relative's home, a simulated apartment, or the community group home(s). Settings within the vocational domain might include the resident's employment setting, work experience job-site, the local sheltered workshop, or competitive job-sites where peers are presently employed. A sample of recreation/leisure environments might include the community parks facilities, YMCA, bowling alleys, movie theaters, spectator sporting events, and the public library. Finally, general community functioning events include such activities such as shopping in supermarkets and department stores, traveling in, out, and around town, and dining in restaurants.

One vehicle for assisting an interview process would be to develop a list that includes several examples of representative settings within domestic, vocational, recreation/leisure and community functioning areas. Table 10.2 contains a sample outline for locating settings in a local community to assist an interview process.

Table 10.2 Survey of Community Environment Frequented by (name of resident)

This survey is a means to find out the frequency of contact *(resident's name)* has with different community settings in the *(community's name)* area. Please fill in the blanks beside the headings where *(resident's name)* goes at least one time a month. After completing the entire form, please place a check mark (✔) in front of those settings where *(resident's name)* has at least weekly contact.

Domestic Areas:
Home: _____
Relative's Home: _____
_____
_____
_____
Friend's Home: _____
_____
_____
Stimulated School Apartment: _____
Other Domestic Settings: _____
_____
_____

Vocational Areas:
Work Setting: _____
Work Experience Settings: _____
_____
_____
_____
_____
Sheltered Workshops: _____
_____
_____
_____
Competitive Job-Sites: _____
_____
_____

Other Vocational
Sites: _____

_____

_____

_____

_____

Recreation/Leisure Areas
Community Parks: _____

_____

_____

_____

Swimming Facilities: _____

_____

_____

_____

Bowling Alleys: _____

_____

_____

_____

Movie Theaters: _____

_____

_____

_____

Spectator
Sporting Events: _____

_____

_____

_____

Other
Recreation Facilities: _____

_____

_____

_____

General Community Functioning Areas
Fast Food
Restaurants: _____

_____

_____

_____

Family Dining
Restaurants: _____
_____
_____
_____
_____

Supermarkets: _____
_____
_____
_____
_____

Department Stores: _____
_____
_____
_____
_____

Usual Mode of
Transportation: _____
_____
_____
_____
_____

Other Community
Environments Not
Included In Other
Categories: _____
_____
_____
_____
_____
_____

Locate Specific Environment

The location of the targeted activity within each of the environments listed in Step 1 is now determined. Using a hand-washing example, the bathrooms within a large mall may be found in several locations. Directions to these bathrooms should be specified for persons who are unfamiliar with these areas and who may be involved in training activities with the resident across each setting. Thus in Figure 10.1 each dissimilar sub-behavior is divided further into features of the bathroom that are most apt to distinguish that bathroom setting from another bathroom setting.

Analyze Characteristics of Activities

As a requirement for this step, it is necessary for the trainer to observe the resident's nonhandicapped peers perform the targeted activity in the settings of Step 1. While observing these peers in natural settings, the trainer should note distinctive subbehaviors of the activity. Each subbehavior also has features that differentiate the way it is uniquely performed in each environment. These distinguishing features should be delineated. Again, using a hand-washing activity as an example, figure 10.1 contains the information described in this section.

For example, a handwashing activity can be divided into four subbehaviors, namely, turning on the cold water, putting soap on the hands, washing hands, and drying hands. Three of these subbehaviors are performed differently depending on the physical features of each bathroom. Only the subbehavior of actually washing the hands is constant across each setting. Thus, in figure 10.1 each dissimilar subbehavior is divided further into features of the bathroom that are most apt to distinguish that bathroom setting from another bathroom setting.

Beneath the subbehavior of turning on the cold water, there are six distinguishing features including: a) the type of faucet handle, b) the location of the cold water faucet, c) the method of grasping the faucet handle, d) the movement required to turn on the cold water, e) the distance the faucet is moved, and f) the movement required to turn off the cold water. There are five task features associated with putting soap on the hands. Specifically, these include: a) the type of soap, b) the location of soap, c) the type of soap dispenser, d) the movement required of H-1 (dominant hand), and e) the movement required of H-2 (nondominant hand). The third subbehavior of handwashing, drying hands, includes six features: a) the type of drying material, b) the location of drying material, c) the method of obtaining the drying material, d) the movement required of H-1 only, e) the movement required of both H-1 and H-2, and f) the type of garbage container.

WASHING HANDS

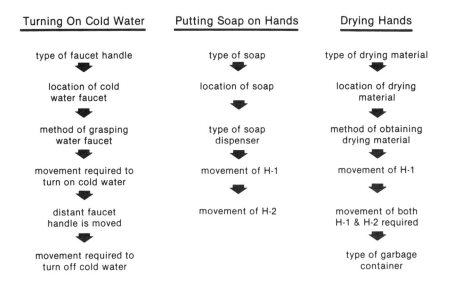

Turning On Cold Water	Putting Soap on Hands	Drying Hands
type of faucet handle	type of soap	type of drying material
location of cold water faucet	location of soap	location of drying material
method of grasping water faucet	type of soap dispenser	method of obtaining drying material
movement required to turn on cold water	movement of H-1	movement of H-1
distant faucet handle is moved	movement of H-2	movement of both H-1 & H-2 required
movement required to turn off cold water		type of garbage container

Fig. 10.1 Subbehavior of Washing Hands

Develop Data Sheets

Figure 10.2 contains a sample data sheet for recording the frequency of a distinguishing feature across activity environments. The letters A-X above each column represent the individual environments where an activity occurs. There is room on the left side of the data sheet to include the subbehavior, the distinguishing features, and the range of each distinguishing feature. For example, the subbehavior of "putting soap on the hands" is written at the top of the left section of the page. Beneath this subbehavior are two of the distinguishing features of putting soap on the hands, namely, "type of soap" and "location of soap dispenser." Beneath each distinguishing feature is the range of that feature.

The range of features for type of soap includes liquid, powdered, or bar varieties. Also, there could be instances when there would be no soap present in a bathroom facility.

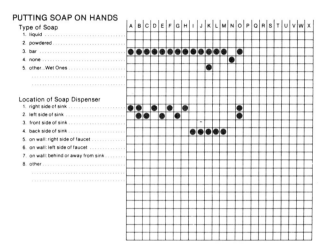

Fig. 10.2

Use Data Sheets in Specific Environments

After constructing the data sheets in step 4, the trainer now returns to all environments in step 2. In these environments the subbehaviors are evaluated by recording the occurrence of a distinguishing feature of that activity. For example, figure 10.2 contains a completed data sheet for fifteen bathrooms that were located in the environments delineated in step 1. As noted on the data sheet, fourteen of the fifteen bathrooms has "wet ones" as well as bar soap. The soap was located in several positions including:a) the right side of the sink (six bathroom), the left side of the sink (five bathrooms), and at the back of the sink (four bathrooms).

Develop Task Analyses

Task analysis refers to the process of dividing a complex behavior into small subcomponents and sequencing these subcomponents in a logical order. The data from the environmental analysis of the handwashing activity provide the information for the development of task analyses for selected bathroom environments. Table 10.3 contains s sample task analyses for a bathroom that contains the distinguishing features of two faucet levers, a bar of soap, and paper towels.

Table 3. Selected Task Analysis of Handwashing Activity

Task Relevant Cue	Response
1. Sink with two faucet levers	1. Using dagger grip, grasp right faucet
2. Hand on the right faucet	2. Turn lever in clockwise direction
3. Lever is being turned in clockwise direction	3. Stop turning lever at less than 90 degree rotation
4. Lever at less than 90 degree rotation	4. Release grasp of faucet lever
5. Cold water coming from spout	5. Place both hands beneath stream of cold water
6. Hands are wet and bar of soap is on basin	6. Pick up soap
7. Soap in hands	7. Rub soap between hands
8. Hands are soapy and bar of soap is in hands	8. Place soap on side of basin
9. Palm of hands are soapy and no bar of soap is in hands	9. Rub palm of each hand over the back of the other hand
10. Entire hands are soapy	10. Place both hands beneath stream of cold water
11. Soapy hands are in stream of cold water	11. Rub palm of each hand over the back of the other hand
12. Hands are wet and no soap is on hands	12. Shake hands over basin to remove excess water from hands
13. Wet hands out of stream of water	13. Using dagger grip, grasp right faucet
14. Dagger grip on right faucet	14. Turn lever in counterclockwise direction
15. No water coming from spout	15. Release grasp of faucet lever
16. Wet hands	16. Locate paper towel dispenser
17. Paper towel dispenser to _____ of sink	17. Using pincer hold, grasp mid-section of single sheet of paper towel
18. Pincer hold on towel sheet	18. Pull down on paper towel

19. Paper towel in H-1 and both hands are wet	19. With paper towel in H-1, rub front and back of H-2
20. Paper towel in H-1 and towel is wet	20. Place paper towel in H-2
21. Paper towel in H-2, and H-1 is wet	21. With paper towel in H-2, rub front and back of H-1
22. Wet towel in hands	22. Locate wastebasket
23. Wastebasket to _____ of sink	23. Drop wet paper towel in wastebasket
24. Hands are still wet	24. Repeat steps 16-22

A unique aspect of writing task analysis in the manner listed in Table 10.2 is the appearance of two columns: one titled "Task Relevant Cue" and the other titled "Response" (Bellamy, Horner, & Inman, 1979) The response column contains the sequence of behaviors the student performs in order to meet the criterion of successfully washing his/her hands. The steps in the first column present the environmental cues that should set the occaision for the corresponding behavior in the response section. for example, when a student sees a sink with two faucet handles (Task Relevant Cue #1), s/he should grasp the right faucet using a dagger-type grip. The sequence of pairing the expected response with a corresponding task relevant cue is very important, especially for conducting baseline assessments and providing cues/correction strategies during training.

Develop Training Strategies

The training strategies recommended in this section are intended to facilitate the generalization of the handwashing behavior to untrained settings. The key element is the choice of the bathroom(s) where concentrated training will occur. Specifically, that bathroom which contains the most common features of all the bathrooms should be the environment of first choice as a training setting.

While training the handwashing behavior in a community bathroom, adherence to the task analyses written in step 6 is of prime importance. The final objective is to have the student respond to the task relevant cue and not to depend on trainer assistance. The trainer's job is to provide the least amount of cues/corrections that still allow the student to complete the response and fade from the external cues/corrections procedures as quickly as possible. A least prompting system is generally advocated as a first strategy toward allowing the student access to information about the required response from a least to most assistance sequence.

Summary

The seven step outline delineated in Table 10.1 does take considerable time to implement. However, if an underlying philosophy for working with residents with severe handicaps is an integration into more normalizing experiences then the effort at enhancing the generalization of skills from home environments to life functioning areas is of extreme importance. By adhering to this outline, a trainer will be developing experiences with a high probability that the acquired skill will generalize to other similar settings, In the past, residential trainers have been content to document in-house progress as an adequate measure of resident achievement. Currently, however, the requirements will begin to be more stringently applied to how well the resident performs in out-of-home-environments. This generalization strategy will provide trainers with a tool to meet the new demands of accountability.

Chapter 11

Characteristics of Model Training Efforts Within Residential Settings

INCLUDED IN this chapter are ten characteristics of quality indicators within residential settings that distinguish model training efforts from less functional systems of program development. Following a description of each characteristic, a self-evaluation checklist is provided to assess a facility's adherence to several levels of each characteristic.

Essential characteristics include:

1. An established philosophy statement
2. A domain referenced curriculum
3. Community-based activities
4. Interaction with nonhandicapped peers
5. Involvement of citizen-advocates/neighbors
6. Systematic instructional strategies with data based decision procedures
7. Hierarchy of documented procedures for a decrease of interferring behaviors.
8. Regular in-service meetings to update staff members on current state-of-the-art information
9. Detailed schedules for each resident
10. Use of generic medical and community services

An Established Philosophy Statement

Each residential facility has overall guiding principles for its operation. One principle common to most facilities is that of normalization. Wolfensberger (1980) provides the following updated definition of normalization:

> The use of means which are culturally normative to offer a person life conditions at least at good as the average citizen's and to as much as possible enhance or support personal behaviors, appearances, status, and reputation to the greatest degree possible at any given time for each individual according to his or her developmental needs. (p 80)

As a cautionary note, the mere fact that a facility has a precise definition of normalization in its charter does not guarantee an operationalized use of this principle (McCord, 1982). Sample questions which help identify facilities that have operationalized the normalization principle are contained in Table 11.1 from Pieper and Cappuccilli (1980).

Additional philosophy principles may also be included in the rationale for residential training programs, including the following:

"Criterion of Ultimate Functioning: the everchanging, expanding, localized, and personalized cluster of factors that each person must possess in order to function as productively and independently as possible in socially, vocationally, and domestically integrated community environment." (Brown, Nietupski, & Hamre-Nietupski, 1976, p. 11)

Dignity of Risk: You are a human being and so you have the right to live as other humans live, even to the point where we will not take all dangers of human life from you (Perske, 1972).

Competence-Deviance Hypothesis: The more competence an individual has, the more deviance will be tolerated in him by others. Deviance = aspects of an individual which cause negative attention and Competence = attributes and skills which not everyone has, and which are appreciated and needed by someone else (Gold, 1980).

"Least Restrictive Environments: Four critical steps toward its implementation. 1) Delineate the current and subsequent environments that are currently available and used in the community of concern...2) Delineate the current and subsequent environments that are used in other communities in the country...3) Delineate the current and subsequent environments which are potentially available and usable in the community... 4) Decide upon, develop, and use the environments that best represent the concept "least restrictive..." (Brown, Branston-McClean, Baumgart, Vincent, Falvey, & Schroeder, 1979, pp. 416-417)

Table 11.1. Questions About Facilities And Their Residents
To Determine If Normalization Is An Operationalized Concept

1. Did the residents choose to live in the home?
2. Is this the type of setting usually inhabited by people in the resident's age group?
3. Do the residents live with others their own age?
4. Is the residence located within a residential neighborhood?
5. Does the residence look like the other dwellings around it?
6. Can the number of people living in the residence be reasonably expected to assimilate into the community?
7. Are community resources and facilities readily accessible from the residence?
8. Do the residents have a chance to buy the house?
9. Do the managers of the place act in an appropriate manner toward the residents?
10. Are the residents encouraged to do all they can for themselves?
11. Are the residents encouraged to use community resources as much as possible?
12. Are all the residents' rights acknowledged?
13. Are the residents being given enough training and assistance to help them be competent, growing, developing individuals?
14. Would I want to live in the home?

Domain Referenced Curriculum

A domain referenced curriculum refers to establishing a sequence of activities and competencies in one of four areas: community mobility, domestic living, recreation leisure and vocational experiences (Brown et al., 1979). Community mobility includes activities such as using public transportation, shopping in supermarkets and department stores, and dining in public restaurants. Domestic living skills are those competencies that are necessary for functioning as independently as possibly within one's place of residence. Sample skills include cooking, mending, laundering, dining, and personal hygiene and grooming. Recreation leisure activities are those events that one engages in to relax, exert physical energy outside of work, or be a spectator at a community event. Finally, the vocational domain refers to the probable or current work settings where a resident is employed and or may be employed. If communication via signing was a targeted skill in a domain referenced curriculum, the signing would occur within the context of one of the domain activities, such as communicating at a meal in the domestic living area. Table 11.2 contains a list of more traditional curriculum headings and how they can be incorporated within the proposed domain areas.

Table 11.2 Translating Traditional Domain to Functional Context

| | DOMAINS | | | |
SKILLS	COMMUNITY MOBILITY	DOMESTIC LIVING	RECREATION LEISURE	VOCATIONAL
SENSORIMOTOR	Walking up a hill or on an uneven sidewalk for balancing.	Adjusting water temperature for a shower or bath.	Tracking a ball to be hit in a game of baseball.	Quality control check for bad parts of an assembled item.
COMMUNICATION	Ordering food at a fast-food restaurant.	Signing wants and needs while at home.	Playing a table game (Bingo) and listening for called numbers.	Talking to customers and coworkers as a busperson.
FINE MOTOR	Putting coins into a vending machine or bus.	Sorting silverware after meal.	Playing cards	Soldering parts on a circuit board.
SELF-CARE	Choosing clothes that correspond to weather for the day.	Morning hygiene routine.	Readying self for an evening out on the town.	Safety behavior while engaging in work task.
SOCIALIZATION	Attending a dance located downtown.	Dinner conversation	Listening to record player and dancing with others.	Small talk during a workbreak.
ACADEMIC	Recognizing names of stores to purchase correct items.	Reading labels of cleaning liquids	Playing table game and moving token appropriate number of spaces.	Signing and cashing check from work.

Community-Based Activities

A general characteristic of severely handicapped individuals is their inability to generalize previously acquired behaviors to new situations (Sailor & Guess, 1983, Snell & Renzaglia, 1987). Stokes and Baer (1977) emphasize the need to program for generalization and not merely expect it to occur by chance; i.e., train and hope. One procedure to ensure the likelihood of generalization to community settings is to conduct most of the training in those community environments where the behaviors are ultimately expected to be performed. For example, if a trainer was teaching a resident how to purchase a movie ticket, s/he could simulate the activity at the residential setting or plan to train the necessary behaviors at an actual theater in the community. Again, there is limited confidence that behaviors learned within the confines of the residential setting would generalize to performance in community environments.

Taking the community training concept a step further, the trainer should be looking for the best example(s) of the community activity thereby limiting the need to train a behavior in all possible settings. Using the ticket purchasing behavior from the previous paragraph, the trainer should analyze the similar and dissimilar methods of purchasing a ticket at all movie theaters within a reasonable proximity. After completing this analysis, s/he should choose the fewest number of theaters that sample the entire range of possibilities for purchasing a ticket and teach those examples to the resident. These analyses were detailed in Chapter 10.

Interaction With Nonhandicapped Peers

Throughout the educational development of severely handicapped students there is a mandate to provide experiences in the least restrictive setting. (P.L. 94-142) One major interpretation of least restrictive settings is the extent to which the handicapped students are involved with nonhandicapped peers throughout the school day (Bates, Renzaglia, & Wehman, 1981; Wilcox & Bellamy, 1982). This interaction with nonhandicapped peers should not abruptly cease when leaving the confines of the school environment. Planned activities must occur to encourage the active involvement of nonhandicapped peers in diverse community events.

Several suggestions are included that facilitate the process of integrating handicapped residents with their nonhandicapped peers:

1. The development of a local chapter of a YARC (Youth Association for Retarded Citizens) whose members actively pursue interactions with severely handicapped residents.
2. Organization of a People First chapter in the area of the residential facility. This organization of handicapped individuals has a prominent goal of getting people on community boards of directors, committees, and positions of power where decisions are made (Edwards, 1982).
3. Students for Exceptional Children (SCEC) may develop a

friend relationship with a handicapped peer who lives in a residential setting.
4. Nonsegregated recreation opportunities should be advocated, i.e., not an all retarded bowling league on Saturday mornings. Activities such as bowling have handicaps attached to the scores. Thus, all participants bowl on an equal basis.
5. Encourage residents to master community mobility skills so a small number can move more independently and participate in community events such as going to the movies, dances, playing bingo, etc.
6. Encourage residents to attend church services on a regular basis and participate in scheduled activities.

Involvement of Citizen-Advocates and Neighbors

Acceptance of a residential facility by community members can be enhanced by the following strategies (Stickney, 1976):
1. upgrade and maintain the facility and its grounds;
2. avoid putting a sign or label on the residence, so that the facility will look the same at its neighbors;
3. provide needed nonresidential services to the community;
4. fill the residence gradually, and introduce residents one-by-one to local services;
5. always try to keep the public informed of the planning group's purposes and program, and do not surprise the neighbors;
6. encourage one-to-one sponsorship of a resident by a community volunteer;
7. establish a program for the residents themselves to serve as volunteers;
8. encourage neighbors' support, not only as volunteers in some aspects of the program, but as donors of items for the home and its residents;
9. create opportunity for the individual residents to meet on social occasions with their new neighbors;
10. start a food cooperative or participate with an existing neighborhood food cooperative;
11. provide adequate supervision of residents, and make sure it is visible to the rest of the community.

When the previous suggestions are adhered to, neighbors can be a valuable asset to the successful functioning of the residential facility (Perske, 1980).

Systematic Instruction Strategies With
Data Based Decision Procedures

Informal interactions often occur between staff members and residents when residents learn new behaviors. However, when a resident fails to acquire a behavior through nonspecific training cues a more formal, systematic approach is needed. Systematic instruction refers to the planned arrangement of antecedent and consequent events with the aim of changing existing behavior. Haring (1977) delineates eight steps of a systematic instructional process.

1. Assessment of general and specific skills.
2. Establishment of long-term objectives or goals for each skills area of behavior of concern.
3. Establishment of and sequencing of short-term objectives (steps leading to each long-term objective).
4. Development and writing of an instruction plan.
5. Development and writing measurement procedures for each behavior.
6. Implementation of the instructional plan and measurement procedures.
7. Modification of the plan based on data.
8. Evaluation of overall pupil progress.

Bates and Pancsofar (1981b) provide a detailed description of strategies for each step in the systematic process. One recommendation is in the sequencing of cues delivered by the trainer. One suggested format is delineated in Figure 7.1 and is known as least prompting. The objective is to provide the resident with the least amount of external assistance in order to occasion a desired response. If this is not powerful enough, an additional, more intense cue is delivered until the desired behavior occurs.

Data based decision making occurs in three phases: baseline, formative, and summative evaluations. During baseline, the trainer's task is to arrange the environment for the resident to respond to the task relevant cues without external assistance (training). During formative assessment, data are collected to assist the trainer in continuing, changing, or discontinuing the present instructional strategies. Finally, during summative assessment the trainer can evaluate the overall success of the interventions and determine if his/her cues and/or reinforcement procedures were responsible for the resultant change in the resident's behavior.

Hierarchy Of Documented Procedures For The Decrease Of Aberrant Behavior

In residential settings for severely handicapped residents, there is an obligation to implement the least intrusive, yet effective, intervention to decrease undesirable behaviors. A process should be in place that delineates the steps to follow ranging from formal to informal means of altering undesirable behaviors both in residential and community settings. One suggested decision model is outlined by Gaylord-Ross (1980). Each component is briefly described in the following sections.

Assessment:
  Is there really a problem?
  Do data substantiate a problem?
  Are there medical explanations?

Reinforcement Procedures:
  Does positive reinforcement for alternative behaviors influence aberrant behavior?
  Are negative reinforcement contingencies effective?
  Is the density of reinforcement sufficent?

Ecological Procedures:
  Is crowding a factor?
  Are there few engaging objects for resident to interact with?
  Are pollutants present?

Task-Specific Procedures:
  Do activities and aberrant behavior covary?
  Are activities too difficult?
  Are activities of low preference value for residents?

Punishment Procedures:
  Are implementation strategies in place for following procedures:
  verbal reprimands, resonse cost, time-out, overcorrection

In addition to the previous considerations for developing strategies to deal with aberrant behaviors, guidelines must be established to insure due process and ethical considerations are accounted for in the residential setting's policy statement regarding the use of intrusive measures to decrease undesirable resident behaviors.

Regular Inservice Sessions to Update Staff on Current State-of-the-Art Knowledge

A licensing requirement by most accreditation agencies is the inclusion of inservice training sessions for residential staff members. The development of a high quality staff is contingent upon members having current knowledge of proven intervention strategies in the field of special education. Monies are appropriated by the federal government for research on model delivery systems for handicapped individuals. To keep current with the dissemination of information from these federal projects as well as current research in the field, staff members should attend quarterly inservice meetings. The following suggestions may also assist in maintaining a knowledgeable and up-to-date staff.

1. Provide travel monies to reimburse staff members attendance at state and/or national professional conference.
2. Subscribe to journals including:
   Journal of The Association for Persons With Severe Handicaps,
   Education and Training of the Mentally Retarded, Mental Retardation
3. Invite experts in the area of community habilitation for the severely handicapped to preside over brainstorming work meeting.
4. Encourage staff to visit other local residential settings and compare diverse training approaches.
5. Maintain a current reference library or have access to a university library of special education materials.

Daily Schedule for Each Resident

The purpose of developing a daily schedule for each resident is to establish an accountability system for program implementation. Individual events are scheduled each day and when staff members complete an activity, they place their initials on the schedule indicating its completion. Numerous interruptions during the day may impede the completion of all scheduled activities but a weekly check can indicate if there is a deficiency in the resident's participation in domestic, community mobility, and/or recreation/leisure pursuits. When a staff member begins a work shift, s/he should consult the daily schedule and apportion time for scheduled resident programs as well as other assigned duties. A sample daily schedule for Steve is presented below:

Usual Monday Schedule

7:00 a.m. Morning routine — *Ernie*
           —Making bed
           —Getting dressed
           —Hygiene procedures
7:45 a.m. Free time until breakfast
8:15 a.m. Breakfast: communication procedure — *all staff*
           Breakfast: proper meal procedures —*all staff*
8:45 a.m. Preparation for workshop — *Ernie*
3:30 p.m. Adult education class — *Linda*
4:30 p.m. Meal preparation — *Connie*
5:30 p.m. Dinner: communication procedure — *all staff*
7:00 p.m. Specialized recreation program — *Recreation staff*
9:45 p.m. Evening hygiene routine — *Tom*

Use of Generic Medical Facilities and Community Services

One avenue for enabling residents to interact with nonhandicapped peers is by frequenting medical and social facilities that nonhandicapped people also use. Residents should be encouraged to be consumers of the same range of services that the general public enjoys (i.e., private physicians, medical specialists, dentists, psychologists). Additionally, residents should be encouraged to participate on an equal basis with peers in recreation activities. For example, there is little need to have a Saturday morning bowling league composed of only handicapped bowlers. In a recreation activity where scores can be adjusted (given handicaps), all can participate on an equal basis during regular bowling hours.

Self-Evaluation Checklist

Included in this section is a guide for evaluating an adherence to each of the characteristics of appropriate training programs that were previously detailed. Each residential facility's staff should conduct a yearly self-evaluation to guide in establishing short- and long-range goals for the operation of the facility. The following self-evaluation is presented as a guide for the establishment of criteria for the adherence to each program characteristic. In developing the sample criteria for the self-evaluation, a general rule of thumb for the 1-4 rating follows:

1. Under no circumstances is this an acceptable criterion for this characteristic.
2. This statement is a currently unacceptable criterion but the intent of the characteristic is being addressed.
3. This statement is a currently acceptable criterion but the conditions within this characteristic need to be the focus for refinement.
4. This statement describes the spirit of the intended narrative definition of the characteristic and should be the eventual goal of the residential facility's staff.

An Established Philosophy Statement

_____ 1. There is no written philosophy of orientation for the general operation of the residential facility.

_____ 2. There is a written philosophy statement but in contradiction to the spirit of model definitions of normalization, criterion of ultimate functioning, and least restrictive environments.

_____ 3. There is a written philosophy statement enunciating goals of normalization, criterion of ultimate functioning and least restrictive environment but operationalization of philosophy is questionable.

_____ 4. There is a clearly written and enunciated philosophy with adherence by direct care staff.

Domain Referenced Curriculum

_____ 1. No activities are centered within a functional domain setting.

_____ 2. Less than half of the activities are centered within a functional domain setting.

_____ 3. More than half of the activities are centered within a functional domain setting.

_____ 4. All training activities occur within the context of the four functional domain categories.

Community-Based Activities

_____ 1. No activities occur within the community.

_____ 2. Less than half of all activities occur within a community setting.

_____ 3. More than half of activities occur within the local community and outside the residential facility.

_____ 4. Community activities are chosen with respect to the

best training exemplars that will increase the probability of actively participating in all available community
settings.

Systematic Instructional Strategies with Data Based Decision Procedures

_____ 1. No structured, systematic strategies occur with any
instructional training program for the residents.

_____ 2. Formal instructional training programs occur but little
attempt is made at a systematic instructional process.

_____ 3. Systematic instructional training programs occur but
data are not collected on its utility.

_____ 4. When formal, more intrusive instructional procedures
are used, careful documentation of its success is noted.

Hierarchy of Documented Procedures for the Decrease of Aberrant Behavior

_____ 1. No systematic approach is adhered to for the behavioral
intervention of unacceptable resident behaviors.

_____ 2. Written procedures exist for behavioral interventions
but they are not individualized for each resident nor
written in a hierarchial manner.

_____ 3. An individual approach is taken with each resident to
decrease unacceptable behavior but a hierarchy of procedures is not observed.

_____ 4. A systematic, written procedure is outlined from less
intensive to more intensive methods to decrease
unacceptable behavior of the residents.

Interaction with Nonhandicapped Peers

_____ 1. No planned for interaction occurs between residents
and nonhandicapped peers.

_____ 2. Interaction occurs between residents and nonhandicapped peers but in a nonplanned and inconsistent
manner.

_____ 3. Two of the six recommendations in the narrative
occur with participation in each activity on at lest a
monthly basis.

_____ 4. Four of the six recommendations in the narrative
occur with participation in each activity on at least a
monthly basis.

Involvement of Citizen-Advocates and/or Neighbors

_____ 1. No intentional, self-initiated contact occurs between
residents and community-advocates/neighbors.

_____ 2. Contact with neighbors occurs but not always on a
pleasant note.

_____ 3. Planned activities occur to involve an interaction between residents and community members but each resident does not have a community-advocate.

_____ 4. An active plan is in operation to encourage residents and neighbors to intereact on at least a monthly basis and a community-advocate is paired with each resident.

Regular In-service Sessions to Update Staff on Current State-of-the-Art Knowledge

_____ 1. No in-service sessions are conducted to update staff on instructional procedures and curriculum development.

_____ 2. In-service sessions are held once a year but lack information of current utility to the staff.

_____ 3. In-service sessions occur four times a year but lack a precise connection to staff members' current work.

_____ 4. In-service sessions occur on a monthly basis to update staff with current state-of-the-art information relative to instructional programs and curriculum development.

Daily Schedule for Each Resident

_____ 1. No daily schedule is evident for any resident.

_____ 2. A general weekly schedule is written for each resident but there is little relationship between the schedule and the residents' current activities.

_____ 3. Daily activity schedules are written for each resident without assignment of the staff who are responsible for its implementation.

_____ 4. Daily schedules are written for each resident with an assignment of a staff person who is responsible for its implementation or an explanation for its nonoccurrence.

Use of General Medical Facilities and Community Services

_____ 1. The providers of all medical and community services are common for all residents.

_____ 2. Medical and community activities occur in segregated and isolated locations within the community.

_____ 3. More than half of activities that residents participate in within the community are their own choice or the choice of an advocate/friend.

_____ 4. Each resident has his/her private doctor, dentist, counselor, etc. who was selected based on the unique needs of the resident and not for mere convenience.

References

Baker, B. L., Seltzer, G. B., & Seltzer, M. M. (1977). *As Close as Possible: Community Residences for Retarded Adults.* Boston Little, Brown and Company.

Baker, D. B. (1979). Severely handicapped: Toward an inclusive definition. *AAESPH Review, 4,* 52-65.

Bates, P. & Barcus, M., eds. (1982). *Curriculum Guide Outline for Community/Vocational Model.* Columbia, SC: Richland County School District One.

Bates, P. & Pancsofar, E., eds. (1979). *A Pictorial Food Preparation Manual: A Cookbook for Training Meal Preparation to Moderately Retarded Students.* Marion IL: Southern Illinois Education Services Center.

Bates, P., & Pancsofar, E. (1981a). *Longitudinal Vocational Training for Severely Handicapped Students in the Public Schools.* Springfield, IL: Illinois State Board of Education, Department of Adult, Vocational and Technical Education/Research and Development Section.

Bates, P., & Pancsofar, E. (1981b). *Program strategies for Preparing Developmentally Disabled Individuals for Community Living.* St. Paul, MN: Bock Associates.

Bates, P., Renzaglia, A., & Wehman, P. (1981). Characteristics of an appropriate education for severely and profoundly handicapped students. *Education and Training of the Mentally Retarded, 16,* 142-149.

Bellamy, G. T., Horner, R. H., & Inman, D. P. (1979). *Vocational Habilitation of Severely Retarded Adults: A Direct Service Technology.* Baltimore, MD: University Park Press.

Billingsley, F. F., & Romer, L. T. (1983). Response prompting and the transfer of stimulus control: Methods, research, and a conceptual framework. *Journal of the Association for the Severely Handicapped, 8*(2), 3-12.

Blatt, B. (1980). Opening remarks at the critical moment. A symposium at the annual convention of the Association for the Severely Handicapped, Los Angeles.

Blatt, B. (1981). *In and Out of Mental Retardation: Essays on Educability, Disability, and Human Policy.* Baltimore: University Park Press.

Bock, W. M., & Weatherman, R. F. (1976). *Minnesota Developmental Programming System, Revised Ed.* Minneapolis, MN: University of Minnesota.

Board of Trustees of The California State University and Colleges. (1978). *Way to Go.* Baltimore: University Park Press, 1978.

Bogdan, R. (1979). *The Community Imperative: A Refutation of all Arguments in Support of Institutionalizing Anybody Because of Mental Retardatioin.* Unpublished paper, Center on Human Policy, Syracuse University.

Bogdan, R., & Taylor, S. (1975). *Introduction to Qualitative Research Methods.* New York: John Wiley.

Bradley, V. J. (1978). *Deinstitutionalization of Developmentally Disabled Persons.* Baltimore: University Park Press

Brown, L., Branston-McClean, M. B., Baumgart, D., Vincent, L., Falvey, M., & Schroeder, J. (1979). Utilizing the characteristics of current and subsequent least restrictive environments in the development of curricular content for severely handicapped students. *AAESPH Review,* 4, 407-424.

Brown, L., Nietupski, J., & Hamre-Nietupski, S. (1976). The criterion of ultimate functioning and public school services for severely handicapped students. In E. Sontag, J. Smith, & N. Certo, eds. *Educational Programming for the Severely and Profoundly Handicapped.* Reston, VA: Council for Exceptional Children.

Buscaglia, L. F. (1982). *Living, Loving and Learning.* New York: Holt, Rinehart and Winston.

Community Services Subcommittee, Deinstitutionalization Task Force. (1983). *Residential Services in Ohio: The Need to Shift from a Facility-Based to a Home-Centered Service System.* Columbus, OH: Ohio Department of Mental Retardation and Developmental Disabilities.

Conley, R. W. (1973). *The Economics of Mental Retardation.* Baltimore, MD: Johns Hopkins University Press.

Dubos, R. (1981). *Celebrations of Life.* St. Louis: McGraw-Hill.

Edgerton, R. B., & Langness, L. L. (1978). Observing mentally retarded perons in community settings: An anthropological perspective. In G. P. Sackett, ed., *Observing Behavior (Vol. 1): Theory and Applications in Mental Retardation.* Baltimore, MD: University Park Press.

Edwards, J. P. (1982). *We are People First: Our Handicaps are Secondary.* Portland, OR: EDNICK, Inc.

Freagon, S., Wheeler, J., Hill, L., Brankin, G., & Costello, D. (1982). *A Domestic Training Environment for Severely Handicapped Students.* Manuscript prepared for a Poster Session at the annual convention of The Association for the Severely Handicapped (TASH). Denver, CO.

Fredericks, B. H. D., Baldwin, V. L., Heyer, M., Romer, L., Romer, M., Gage, M. A., Vladimiroff, L., & Johnson, N. (1979). Community living skills: Curriculum, clients, and trainers. In G. T. Bellamy, G. O'Connor, & O. C. Karan, eds. *Vocational Rehabilitation of Severely Handicapped Persons: Contemporary Service Strategies* (pp. 229-252) Baltimore:University Park Press

Gage, M. A., Fredericks, H. B., Baldwin, V. L., Moore, W. G., & Grove, D. (1977). An alternative pattern of educational/residential care and services for mentally retarded children. *AAESPH Review, 2,* 146-156.

Gardner, J. M. (1977). Community residential alternatives for the developmentally disabled. *Mental Retardation,* 15(6), 3-8.

Gaylord-Ross, R. (1980). A decision model for the treatment of aberrant behavior in applied settings. In W. Sailor, B. Wilcox, & Brown, eds. *Methods of Instruction for Severely Handicapped Students.* Baltimore: Paul H. Brookes.

Gold, M. W. (1980). *Marc Gold: "Did I Say That?" Articles and Commendary on the Try Another Way System.* Champaign, IL: Research Press.

Gollay, E., Freedman, R., Wyngaarden, M., & Kurtz, N. R. (1978). *Coming back: The Community Experiences of Deinstitutionalized Mentally Retarded People.* Cambridge, MA: Abt Associates.

Gross, A. M. (1977). The use of cost effectiveness analysis in deciding on alternative living environments for the retarded. In P. Mittler, ed. *Research to Practice in Mental Retardation: Care and Intervention, Vol. 1.* (pp. 427-433) Baltimore, MD: University Park Press.

Gunzberg, H. C. (1974). *Progress Assessment Chart of Social and Personal Development: Manual (3rd ed.).* Birmingham, England: SEFA Ltd.

Halle, J., Marshall, A., & Spradlin, J. E. (1979). Time delay: A technique to increase language usage and facilitate generalization in retarded children. *Journal of Applied Behavior Analysis, 12,* 341-349.

Haring, N., ed. (1977). *The Experimental Education Training Program—An Inservice Program for Personnel Serving the Severely Handicapped.* Seattle: University of Washington.

Heal, L. W., & Daniels, B. S. (1978). *A Cost-Effectiveness Analysis of Residential Alternatives for Selected Developmentally Disabled Citizens of Three Northern Wisconsin Counties.* Denver, CO: Annual meeting of the American Association on Mental Deficiency.

Heal, L. W., & Laidlaw, T. J. (1980). Evaluation of residential alternatives. In A. R. Novak & L. W. Heal, eds. *Integration of Developmentally Disabled Individuals into The Community.* Baltimore, MD: Paul H. Brookes.

Heal, L. W., Novak, A. R., Sigelman, C. K., & Switzky, H. N. (1980). Characteristics of community residential facilities. In A. R. Novak & L. W. Heal, eds. *Integration of Developmentally Disabled Individuals into the Community* (pp. 45-56) Baltimore: Paul H. Brookes.

Howse, J. L. (1980). Piecing together existing financial resources. In P. Roos, B. M. McCann & M. R. Addison, eds. *Shaping the Future: Community-Based Residential Services and Facilities for Mentally Retarded People.* Baltimore, MD: University Park Press.

Hungerford, R. H. (1950). On locusts. *American Journal of Mental Deficiency, 54,* 415-418.

Intagliata, J. C., Willer, B.S., & Cooley, F.B. (1979). Cost Comparison of institutionalized and community based alternatives for mentally retarded persons. *Mental Retardation, 17,* 134-136.

Jones, P. P., & Jones, J. J. (1976). *Cost of Ideal Services to the Developmentally*

Disabled Under Varying Levels of Adequacy (Interim report #4, HEW Contract OS-74-278). Medford, MA: Florence Heller School, Brandeis University.

Kazdin, A. E. (1980). *Behavior Modification in Applied Settings.* Homewood, IL: Dorsey Press.

Laski, F. (1980). The right to live in the community: The legal foundation. In P. Roos, B. M. McCann, & M. R. Addison, eds. *Shaping the Future: Community-Based Residential Services and Facilities for Menatlly Retarded People* (pp. 151-162) Baltimore: University Park Press.

Lensink, B. R. (1980). Establishing programs and services in an accountable system. IN P. Roos, B. M. McCann & M. R. Addison, eds. *Shaping the Future: Community-Based Residential Services and Facilities for Mentally Retarded People* (pp. 49-66) Baltimore University Park Press.

McCord, W. T. (1982). From theory to reality: Obstacles to the implementation of the normalization principle in human services. *Mental Retardation, 20,* 247-253.

Michell, J. (1981). The ideal world-view. In S. Kumar, ed. *The Schumacher lectures.* New York: Harper Colophon.

Mickenberg, N. H. (1980). A decade of deinstitutionalization: Emerging legal theories and strategies. *Amicus, 5,* 54-63.

Nihira, K., Foster, R., Shellhaas, M., & Leland, H. (1974). *AAMD adaptive Behavior Scale* (1974 revision). Washington, D.C.: American Association on Mental Deficiency.

Nirje, B. (1977). Tenets of normalization. In Canadian Association for the Mentally Retarded, *Orientation Manual on Mental Retardation.* Toronto: National Institute on Mental Retardation.

O'Connor, G. (1976). *Home is a Good Place: A National Perspective of Community Residential Facilities for the Mentally Retarded.* Washington, D. C.: American Association on Mental Deficiency.

Pancsofar, E. (1982. A strategy for teaching severely handicapped students to transfer skills to untrained settings: An environmental and task analysis approach. In S. Maurer, P. Bates, A. Ford, J. Nietupski, J. Nisbet, E. Pancsofar, & S. Teas, eds. *Project A.M.E.S. (Actualization of Mainstream Experience Skills) Vol. 3:* 1981-1982. Des Moines, IA: Department of Public Instruction.

Peat, Marwick, Mitchell, & Company. (1977) *Community Living Alternatives for Persons with Developmental Disabilities. Vol. 1: Financial requirements.* Springfield, IL: Governor's Planning Council on Developmental Disabilities.

Perske, R. (1972). The dignity of risk and the mentally retarded. *Mental Retardation, 10*(1), 24-27.

Perske, R. P. (1980). *New Life in the Neighborhood: How Persons with Retardation or Other Disabilities Can Help Make a Good Community Better.* Nashville, TN: Partheon.

Pieper, B., & Cappuccilli, J. (1980). Beyond the family and the institution: The sanctity of liberty. In T. Apolloni, J. Cappuccilli, & T. P. Cooke eds. *Achievements in Residential Services for Persons with Disabilities: Toward Excellence.* Baltimore: University Park Press.

Rossi, P. H., Freeman, H. E., & Wright, S. R. (1979). *Evaluation: A Systematic Approach*. Beverly Hills, CA: Saga Publications.

Russell, R. D. (1976). *Health Education*. Washington, D.C.: National Education Association.

Sailor, W., & Guess, D. (1983). *Severely Handicapped Students: An Instructional Design*. Boston: Houghton Mifflin.

Scheerenberger, R. C. (1978). *Public Residential Services for the Mentally Retarded*. Madison, WI: National Association of Superintendents of Public Residential Facilities for the Mentally Retarded, Central Wisconsin Center for the Developmentally Disabled.

Snell, M. E. (1982). Analysis of time delay procedures for teaching daily living skills to retarded adults. *Analysis and Intervention in Developmental Disabilities, 2,* 139-155.

Snell, M. E. & Gast, D. L. (1981). Applying time delay procedures to the instruction of the severely handicapped. *Journal of the Association for the Severely Handicapped, 6*(3), 3-14.

Snell, M. E., & Renzaglia, A. M. (1982). Moderate, severe, and profound handicaps. In N. G. Haring, ed. *Exceptional Children and Youth (3rd ed.)* (pp. 143-170). Columbus, OH: Charles E. Merrill.

Stickney, P. (1976). Strategies for gaining community acceptance of residential alternatives. In P. Stickney, ed. *Gaining Community Acceptance: A Handbook for Community Residence Planners*. White Plains, NY: Westchester Community Service Council.

Stokes, T. R., & Baer, D. M. (1977). An implicit technology of generalization. *Journal of Applied Behavior Analysis, 10,* 341-367.

Taylor, S. J., & Bogdan, R. (1981). A qualitative approach to the study of community adjustment. In R. H. Bruininks, C. E. Meyers, B. B. Sigford, & K. C. Lakin, eds. *Deinstitutionalization and Community Adjustment of Mentally Retarded People.* (pp. 71-81). Washington, D.C.: American Association on Mental Deficiency.

Thompson, M. M. (1977). *Housing for the Handicapped and Disabled: A Guide for Local Action*. Washington, D. C.: The National Association of Housing and Redevelopment Officials.

Index